Insig...

And

Guidance

For Spiritual

Seekers

By

Rudra Shivananda

Alight Publications

2009

Insight And Guidance For Spiritual Seekers

By Rudra Shivananda

First Edition Published in July 2009

Alight Publications
PO Box 930
Union City, CA 94587

http://www.Alightbooks.com

ISBN 1-931833-34-6

Printed in the United States of America

Dedicated

to the

Eternal Friend

That Guides
All of Us

Insight and Guidance for Spiritual Seekers

Contents

A Note to the Reader

Part 3: Autumn

Part 4: Winter

Part 5: Renewal

A Note to the Reader

In my travels to distant lands to give the teachings and practices of the ancient science of Self-Realization, I've encountered many diverse spiritual seekers who are in need of positive guidance. Many of them make good use of contemporary communication methods such as email to satisfy their doubts and queries, but it is never enough to quench their spiritual thirst.

Most of the obstacles that appear on the spiritual path are common to sincere seekers and so are the helpful guidance and insights. In order to provide the inspiration that is required, I began to write a regular spiritual journal that was freely emailed to the students. This is called Sanatana Mitra (The Eternal Friend), in honor of the divine Master of Masters called Babaji.

Based on the positive feedback, I've decided to include the recent articles in one volume in order to reach a wider group that may wish to be inspired and aided on their spiritual journey. The themes of these articles are very contemporary and based on recent events or queries from students. I've strived to make all of these articles free from a narrow interpretation of the timeless truths of yoga and so they are applicable to all seekers irrespective of their specific path. There are also practical techniques included because some of the problems on the path are best overcome by simple postures, breathing, meditation or energetic redistribution.

The articles themselves are each only a few pages long in order to reach the specific aspects of the insight quickly – this seems to be necessary in the current rapidly evolving and fast-paced society. It is possible to read these articles in any order as well as in the sequence that they are placed.

My best wishes to you on your spiritual quest. May you persevere and reach your goal.

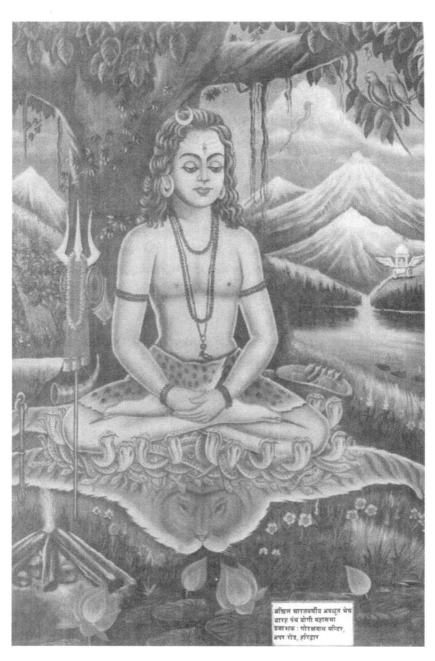

I bow to the Divine MahaGuru Babaji

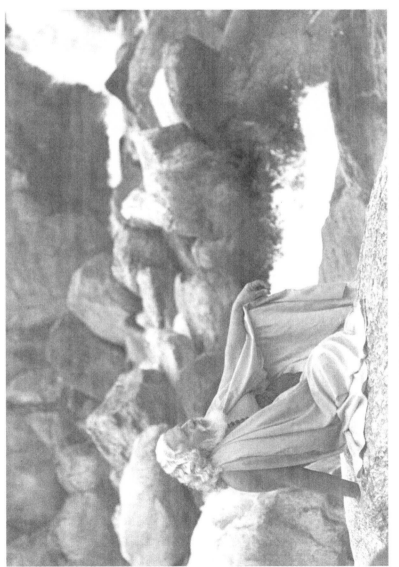

I bow to my Master Yogiraj Gurunath Siddhanath

Transcendental Knowledge Destroys Karma

Knowledge of reality beyond the five senses is termed transcendental. We must understand that by knowledge we should not think of some sort of theoretical information acquired from external sources but rather a direct experience of truth that permanently transforms our framework and perception of reality.

A direct experience of truth transcends the mundane mind that is bound by the five senses and utilizes the intellect or intuitive mind or even the super-mind. Normal mode of speech confuses the intellect with the mundane mind such that the word intelligence is used to mean an acumen in sorting through the miasmic three-dimensional model produced by the five senses. The actual intellect that we are referring to is a higher function of our consciousness and is different from the analytically bound mundane mind.

It is important to realize that we possess higher functions in our consciousness that we are not tapping into systematically or willfully. This is analogous to having access to an electron microscope and limiting oneself to a magnifying glass to examine the complexities of cell structure - it sounds absurd but everyday seekers of truth courageously but foolishly use their sense-bound minds to try to examine reality which is beyond the three dimensions bounded by the five senses.

Karma is the law of cause and effect that manifests in our limited understanding of reality in the guise of reward and punishment and ultimately in the cycle of death and re-birth called re-incarnation. Even though we can understand and wish to believe that positive or "good" actions give rise to a better life in the future and that negative or "bad" actions give rise to a worse

1

future, we cannot perceive the direct relationships between what will happen in some future live and what we are doing now.

When we have experienced reality and have access to transcendental knowledge then we can fully examine the *karmic* process and in doing so have the ability to remove the potential pitfalls that are waiting to befall the three dimensional being and essentially put a stop to the operation of this process.

Therefore one view of the goal of Yoga is the realization of transcendental knowledge which would free one from the operation of Karma and lead to liberation from the cycle of re-birth. This is a desired goal because every birth has its load of suffering (and enjoyment) and will lead to further entanglements in non-reality.

The ancient sages have examined many possible methods of achieving this transcendental knowledge and have selected a small number to be practiced by humanity. The specific path followed by a seeker of truth depends on his or her tendencies in this life towards the various methods blessed by the experiences of those who have successfully achieved their goals and stayed behind to guide their fellow seekers.

The path of selfless work is highly recommended for those who enjoy helping others and revel in activities. They devote themselves to good work and offer the results of their work to the Divine, taking no credit for their actions and therefore taking no negative *karma* either. Sustained effort in this manner leads to the purification of the mundane mind and access to the higher intellectual mind with its consequent effortless direct experience of reality. The path of good works is not focused on higher consciousness or on the experience of reality, only in performing one's work without attachment.

For those who have great faith in the love and power of the Divine, the path of spiritual devotion can remove all the egocentric obstacles to the transcendental experience. Immersion in an image of the Divine and constant prayer leave no room for doubt and selfish activities. The goal is to experience that aspect of the Divine that is the object of devotion.

Then there are the other yogic disciplines such as Hatha Yoga, Raja Yoga, Jnana Yoga and Kriya Yoga, involving rigorous physical /vital and / or mental control in order to storm the citadel of sensory mind and defeat the usurper Lord Ego to directly experience the transcendental reality. These are fast evolutionary paths that require much time and effort but yield proven results in one life-time, as testified by the successful practitioners over many generations.

Rarely, we are blessed with someone who is born with the gift of direct experience of reality. Such a one becomes a beacon of light to show the way and as a testament to our inherent birthright to experience beyond the limitations of the three dimensional playground.

The awareness and experience of reality can be blissful but also disorienting to our previous erroneous physical, emotional and mental conditionings and can lead to periods of eccentric behavior....eccentric to those imprisoned in their limited egocentric world-view.

There are also different levels and intensities of transcendental experience. Sometimes, one may only have a glimpse and spend a whole lifetime trying to integrate it into one's life – this is usually the case of one who is not following a yogic discipline. More often, transcendental experiences follow one another in an escalating series that lead to complete awakening to reality of the Here and Now, to the essence of Being.

During the period of awakening there is both an internalization and externalizing of the experiences to distill them into transcendental knowledge. An analogy would be the application of Einstein's discovery that mass can be converted to energy leading to the production of a nuclear power station to generate electricity. Transcendental knowledge gained from the repeated experience of reality enables the re-wiring of the body-mind complex burning away the *karmic* bonds and restraints and enabling the performance of actions from the perspective of higher dimensional awareness. Actions initiated from the perspective of transcendental knowledge are not subject to the three-dimensional *karmic* laws and instead are synchronized with the laws of higher dimensions.

Ignorance is the Root of Suffering

We often wonder why we suffer. Although in the ultimate sense, we do not know why or how suffering originated, it is possible for enlightened Sages and realized Masters to perceive the process of suffering, pain and sorrow and explain it to us within the realm of the senses.

From their experience of reality, the wise have realized that the root cause of our suffering is ignorance or *avidya*. This is explained as confusing what is unreal as real and what is impermanent with that which is permanent. How does this apply in our limited perspective?

We live our lives as if it will last forever, although the only certainty from birth is death. Nothing else is certain. Yet, we avoid thinking about death until or unless some event intrudes into our self-imposed delusion. Perhaps the passing of a dear one or our own serious illness temporarily will awaken our sense of mortality, but most often we forget again until old age.

Nothing in our experience is permanent. Happiness comes and goes and so does grief. We wish to hold on to the moments of happiness but they slip away – we are powerless to control our emotions. We are powerless to control our thoughts, yet we act as if we are the kings of our own realm and can control our destiny.

We seek permanence in relationships that are based on mutual needs or desires that shift beneath us like mounds of quicksand. In this life, relationships change or are broken and new ones take their place in a rollercoaster ride of love and happiness followed by hate and grief. Our loved ones in this life may become our bitterest enemies in the next – who has control over their relationships?

We seek permanence in possessions that become old or broken, that become stolen or lost and that we cannot take with us into the next world. At what cost have we hoarded our precious trinkets only to see them slip away if not in this life, then the next? People become chained by their possessions and lose their freedom to follow spiritual guidance.

The rich have fear of losing their wealth and think everyone is trying to take their money or possessions. They have to sleep with one eye open to guard their treasures and so suffer greatly. However, this suffering can also occur in the poor – one who has only few possessions but become attached and obsessed with them will be afraid of losing even such trivial objects.

We seek permanence in the physical body which decays and dies. One of the main manifestations of ignorance is the identification of the self with the body. Our five senses give us nothing beyond the body and so our ego sticks us with the infantile notion that we are nothing beyond the body. When the body becomes sick, we say, "I am sick," and we feel terrible. When the body becomes old, we whine, "I am old." In this way, we seek to find happiness through the body, through the senses, but it is always fleeting and we are left thirsty and dissatisfied to the grave.

The identification with the body is so deep that when a part of the body is damaged we feel ourselves as damaged. But, are we the broken arm or leg or even the missing finger? Wisdom passed down from the sages tell us that the body is only a temporary vehicle for the self and is replaced after a lifetime of use, just as our clothing for the physical body is temporary and can be changed.

We seek permanence in the mundane mind that cannot know reality and is only fed data streams from the five senses. This mind limits us to a three dimensional view of reality and it is not even subject to our control, but harbors deep automatic reactions from the subconscious portion of itself. Yet, a second manifestation of ignorance is the identification of the self with the mind. This causes great misery because even though you seldom have control over your thoughts, you identify with the negative thoughts that arise and consequently feel guilt and betrayal by your own mind. If one starts to fear or hate one's own mind then one will hide from self-study or understanding of one's mental processes and therefore not realize the relationship of the limited mind and the self.

Most people also suffer from identification with their emotions and cannot separate their thoughts and emotions from their true self. Fear, rage, lust and a myriad other emotions come and go and we become hostage to the emotion of the moment.

Most people go through life clinging to the promise that there is something permanent -- perhaps the hope of eternal salvation for the eternal soul in an eternal heaven. However, in the spirit of ignorance, they would like to belief that the Divine will resurrect their long decayed physical bodies as well – the rationale for burial of the body!

A small but growing number of seekers after truth have resolved to realize the truth for themselves – to experience reality and freedom from ignorance. They understand that the sages have taught that only the True Self is permanent and so have made Self-Realization their goal in life. They seek the realization that they are not the body or the mind but the eternal Spirit, the True Self. Let us all be seekers of truth and throw off our ignorance by the determined practice of Yoga.

Eternal Friend

O Divine, You are my Eternal Friend.
Let me see You daily in the life-giving Sun and in the Moon
that lights my path in darkness of night.
Let me see You in the tree that gives me shade in blaze of day
and in the fragrant flower that opens briefly in hidden night.

O Divine, You are my Eternal Friend.
Let me hear You in creation's roar that vibrates in every atom
of material manifestation and in mystic mantras bestowed by
blessings of enlightened sages.
Let me hear You in the manic roar of a speeding car through a
quiet neighborhood and in the loud modern music blaring from
boom-boxes or intimately from personal ipods.

O Divine, You are my Eternal Friend.
Let me receive Your grace and perceive Your guidance through
the words of Masters past and living.
Let me receive Your grace and perceive Your guidance through
the words of friends known and unknown.
Let me receive Your grace and perceive Your guidance through
the purified portals of the five senses.
Let me receive Your grace and perceive Your guidance in the
silence of solitude in the depths of my heart.

Focus on Asana –
Camel Pose (Uttrasana)

The Camel Pose is relatively simple but has profound effect on the whole body as it tones the whole spine as well as the chest and abdominal areas while stimulating the endocrine glands. Those who have spondylitis of any potion of the spine can definitely benefit from regular practice of this posture, as can those with diabetes or thryorid /parathyroid disorders.

Kneel with thighs and truck erect, knees slightly apart and hands on the hip.   Reach back as you exhale and arch you back to grab the heels with the hands.   Push buttocks and abdomen forward, arching the back more and bending the head back slowly. Maintain this position with normal breathe for one to three minutes and then return to the original position. Bend the knees and sit on the heels. Slowly exhale and bend forward to rest the forehead on the floor. Relax.

If the previous instructions are too strenuous, use a variation: try leaning back and placing both hand on the buttocks to support yourself, instead of reaching for the heels. Focus your attention on the navel energy center, and breathing naturally.

Refer figure 1 for illustrations of the camel pose.

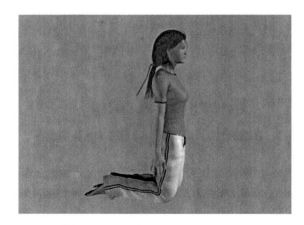

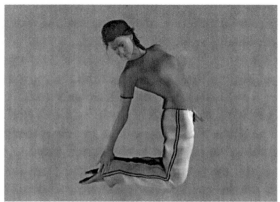

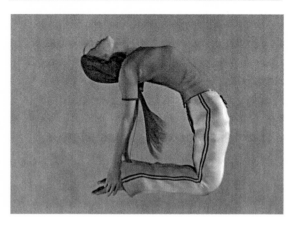

Figure 1: Camel Pose

Accomplishing One's Goal
Without Attachment

As I've been watching the Democratic Party Primaries to determine their candidate for the presidency, it is quite apparent that the Clinton's have great attachment to winning the elections at all cost. To many people this may even be an admirable trait – in fact, it has become very "American" to focus on the goal and forget the process – never mind lying and compromising every principle of decency.

This focus on the desired objective above all other considerations has permeated into sports, business and politics.

But is this really the only way to accomplish one's goals? The wise who have accomplished much would say that it is not necessary to be so attached to one's goals that one must betray one's humanity. Without attachment to the results, one can focus on accomplishing the goal with even greater determination and less stress and fear.

The driving fear is that if one keeps to integrity and higher virtues such as truth and fair-play, one cannot possibly accomplish one's goals. However, history teaches the opposite – time and again, those who strive without virtue may achieve their desires in the short-term but will be undone with time. These "winners" will be vilified. Those who strive in virtue will be honored even if they may have appeared to have lost some contest.

In recent times, look at the case of Al Gore who will be better treated by history than the winner of the political contest. How about the lady athlete who had to give back all of her Olympic gold medals after being convicted of using illegal steroids? We must remember that the end does not justify the means.

I'm reminded of something said by Gandhi, the great soul who helped to bring about the independence of India by the principles of non-violence and truth:

He who is ever brooding over the result, often loses nerve in the performance of duty. He becomes impatient and then gives vent to anger and begins to do unworthy things; he jumps from action to action, never remaining faithful to any. He who broods over results is like a man given to the objects of the senses; he is ever distracted, he says good-bye to all scruples, everything is right in his estimation and he therefore resorts to means fair and foul to attain his end.

Gandhi never brooded over the results – he learned to be detached from them as he was detached even from the sufferings of his body, as he was beaten and imprisoned time and again. Let us accomplish our goals with dedication and keeping the integrity of our values.

Faith, Reason And Experience

Faith is a very much misunderstood word both to those who champion or invoke it and by those who oppose it.

The word has become associated with religion and in fact people popularly say, "Christian Faith," or ask "what is your faith?"

It is ridiculed by rational people who associate it with belief in something or someone against all reason and therefore it is "blind faith."

Voltaire satirized both faith and religion when he defined faith as in believing in the irrational and a Christian as one who continues to subscribe to such faith in the face of all contrary facts and experience.

Why then do we wish to say something positive about faith? It is because the right kind of faith is essential on the spiritual path. Let us not forget that everyday, our experience and reason give us the faith that when we go to sleep we will wake up alive and essentially the same person in the morning. We need to step back and re-examine the negative concepts piled on this word, so that we can understand its rightful place as taught by the spiritual Masters and Yogis.

We may have a belief such as the premise that 'the sun revolves around the earth,' or that, 'there are other life-forms in the Universe.' The first is supported by experience, since we do not feel that the earth moves but the sun appears to move in the sky everyday. Reason would suggest that if the earth was moving, we would feel the movement. Faith in the experience and reason expect that the movements of the planets could be accurately predicted by using the earth-centric model. However, when the model failed to provide the results required, while a sun-centric model did, then experience from the failed model should lead to the reasoning that the belief in an earth-centric model was flawed. Therefore faith should be placed on the sun-centric model.

This example would lead one to analogize that a belief is like a scientific hypothesis and needs to be tested by experience and reason, that is, experiment. Scientists spend many years in experiments to test their hypothesis and when the experiments are positive, then the hypothesis is upgraded to a theory, just as a supported belief becomes faith. When a theory withstands all experiment and attempts to disprove it, as well as has demonstrated the capability to predict events, it becomes a law. Here, the analogy should not be taken too far, but is still somewhat applicable, as a law is a provable scientific statement of reality, while if a person of faith performs certain spiritual experiments on herself, she should be able to demonstrate her attainment in her life.

Let us examine the second example of a belief, that, 'there is life in the Universe, other than on Earth.' Now, reason would dictate that if there were other forms of life we would have met them by now and since we haven't they don't exist. The belief in other life forms persists in scientific circles in spite of the lack of experiential or rational support. The good news is that recently, they have started to discover 'other planets' which then gave rational support to the reasoning that if there are other planets and there may be very many of them, surely some of them would support life-forms. It is interesting to note that the belief for life-forms remained throughout the period when science could not detect any planet, but there was this second belief that there must be other planets. It took many years and a lot of effort to prove that there were other planets. Has the belief that life exist on other planets now become a faith that can drive further activity? It would seem so.

When we venture into the spiritual realm and seek to discover our own place in the Universe or answers to questions such as 'why are we here?', we are entering into a realm where science stops and goes no further.

This discussion on faith now becomes relevant because without faith we cannot attain to the answers we seek, just as their faith sustained the scientists looking for planets in other solar systems. We need to have faith in ourselves, that we are capable of much more than we are displaying right now.

We must have faith in the path we are following. In order to develop this faith, we must test the path with reason and experience. There is no place for 'blind faith' on the spiritual path of yoga.

A spiritual path is a series of experiments performed over time subjectively which will lead to a realization of both the subjective and objective worlds. There is generally one or more founders of this path and we need to test them with reason and experience. If they are still alive, we need to "check them out." If they have passed away, check out their representatives – have they attained to the goals of the path?

What about the person who is transmitting the path to you? Not everyone transmitting the path may have attained to the goal. Does she pass the test? Are there others in the present or past who can testify to the path? Only after a thorough investigation should one place one's faith on the prospective path. After all, before one would drive a particular route from one place to another, one may ask those who have driven by different ways for their recommendations, and/or check the authorized maps given by the experts etc. before proceeding.

Once we have faith on the path, then we can persevere in our efforts to attain to the requisite realization. Without faith, we would give up after some time, before realization can occur. This would be like taking a stop and letting our doubts make us turn back on our drive to our destination.

Sometimes, despite our best efforts, we may be in error on our faith, and we must not abandon all reason and experience, should this be the case. A misplaced faith should be discarded when there is overwhelming evidence against it and an effort made to discover a new path.

Have faith and persevere. Discard doubt, but not experience and reason until the path is won.

Happiness

Clear skies, sunny day
I'm happy, sunlight and life.
Clouds roll in, pouring rain
I'm happy, cooling breeze.

Job well-done, praise comes
I'm happy, Divine work fun.
Blame comes, results disappoint
I'm happy, best effort done.

Best friend, enjoyed the company
I'm happy, positive relationship.
Former friend, slander and lies
I'm happy, space to forgive.

Profit payment, useful tool
I'm happy, purpose fulfilled.
Sudden loss, painful lesson
I'm happy, learn detachment.

Body weak, life draws to close
I'm happy, new beginning.
Spirit soars, now winged delight
I'm happy, Divine light bring.

Non-Attachment

It is taught by the wise that attachment causes unhappiness in life and that the practice of non-attachment is necessary for spiritual development.

We do not frequently examine our attachments nor consider them in a negative light for it is taken for granted that a major goal of life must be to experience pleasure and we are therefore attracted to activities that may satisfy the craving for pleasure. It is through the five senses that we derive most of our pleasures and so we are attached to the sensations from the five senses. The senses depend on the body and mind because the sensory organs are in the body and the mind processes the sensory input to give the experience of pleasure – we are therefore also attached to the body and mind.

When we see someone or something that we are attracted to we form an attachment to it and would like to repeat that experience and so a desire appears in our minds. Desires multiply without limit as we become immersed in the senses. Memories of pleasurable experiences become attached to the desires and our thoughts gravitate towards the gratification of the desires. As we give our desires more and more importance, our thoughts, words and actions rotate around our desires as our earth rotates around the sun.

We can form an attraction to any sensory input from any one or combination of sense organs. We can therefore form a desire from something seen, heard, smelled, touched or tasted. The attraction to a particular type of food might involve the visual aspect, the taste and smell, as well as the texture (touch).

When we are unable to satisfy a desire or our attempts to satisfy a desire is thwarted, the emotion of anger arises. We become angry and strike out at everyone around us. We also become angry with ourselves for the failure to gratify ourselves. Anger becomes an automatic reaction to the inability to satisfy a desire and so we oscillate between desire, satisfaction or pleasure and anger, sometimes spending much more time and energy in the desire and anger phases then in the actual enjoyment phase.

In fact, sometimes, even during the enjoyment phase, the desire for a repetition of the pleasure might arise already and then the emotion of fear rears its uninvited head. There is fear that the pleasure will not come again and therefore this might be the last time the desire is satisfied, or fear that the pleasure will be less next time around. This forms a complex emotional / mental reaction or habit pattern of desire, pleasure, fear and anger.

The reaction pattern of desire, pleasure, fear and anger causes stress and unhappiness. The physical, energetic, emotional and mental health of a person suffers from the stress induced by the attraction and attachment. A person becomes free from tension when there are no desires. Stress and tension leads to the tendency towards ill-health as the body and mind are more susceptible to physical, emotion and mental disease agents.

Desires impact not only ourselves but can have significant effect on others and may even alter the fortunes of countries and the whole world. Many stories have illustrated the impact of desires. A notable Indian epic, the Ramayana is replete with examples – the desire of Rama's step-mother to usurp the kingdom for her own offspring led to the untimely death of her husband and untold hardship for the people of the country. The desire of Sita, Rama's wife for the golden deer led her to send her brother-in-law and protector away, resulting in her being kidnapped by Ravana, the demon-king of Lanka. The desire of Ravana to possess Sita, led to a great war, resulting in his own death and the death of countless heroes. Another epic, the Greek Iliad, recounts how the desires of Paris and Helen for each other, led to the great Trojan War that lasted for ten years.

On smaller scale, the attachment to form has led to girls starving themselves or developing eating disorders. The attachment to relationships has led to the suicides of discarded partners. The attachment to one's ideologies has led to terror bombings and other heinous acts.

Desires are a fact of life. What can you do with them? There are at least three ways of dealing with them – one can satisfy them, one can repress them or one can detach from them. Trying to satisfy our desires is like trying to chop off the head of the mythical monster with many heads – whenever you cut one head off, several appear to take its place. There is not enough time in a lifetime to satisfy all our desires. Repressing our desires only deepen their hold on us – we spend all our time thinking about them, even fantasizing about them, and sooner or later, they will burst forth uncontrollably, causing all sorts of damage. The method recommended by those who have wisdom is to detach from them, to let them pass by without focusing your energy on them. The practice of detachment is extremely difficult but the only one of the three that can lead to happiness, and extrication from the cycle of desire, pleasure, fear and anger.

The practice of detachment is essential for those on the path of spiritual evolution as well as for those who wish to be happy in this life and enjoy good health and long life. One way of detachment is to offer the fruits or results of one's actions to the greater good of humanity, or to the Divine Principle of the Universe etc., something greater than our ego-selves. In this way, we are not attached to the results whether pleasurable or painful and yet be able to enjoy them.

Please do give a little thought to how our attachments are affecting our lives – this will increase our awareness in all our thoughts, words and deeds.

Focus on Pranayama - Prana Mudra

A tonic to awaken and distribute healing energy throughout the body and for releasing physical, emotional and mental blockages. It establishes equanimity and connectedness to the universal source of all energy. This technique is best practiced at sunrise, preferably, facing the sun.

1. Sit in one of the recommended postures, preferably *siddhasana*. Place the right palm on top of the left palm. Close the eyes and relax the whole body, yet maintaining a straight back.
2. Utilizing abdominal breathing, inhale and exhale deeply, expelling the maximum amount of air from the lungs, by contracting the abdominal muscles. While the breath is held out for a moment, contract the perineum and the anal sphincter.
3. While maintaining the contraction of the perineum, begin inhaling slowly, expanding the abdomen fully to draw in the maximum air into the lungs. At the same time, raise the hands to the level of the navel center. The hands are not touching, with fingers pointing towards each other and the palms facing inwards. There should be no tension in the arms. During the inhalation, feel and visualize the *prana* or life-force being drawn from the first energy center or *chakra* to the navel *chakra* along the spinal column.
4. Continue with thoracic breathing, expanding the chest and simultaneously raising the hands to the heart center. Feel the *prana* rising from the navel to the heart along the spine.
5. Complete the inhalation with clavicular breathing, raising the shoulders slightly and drawing some more air into

the lungs. Feel the life-force energy being drawn from the heart center to the throat center, as you raise your hands to the front of the throat.

6. Retain the breath for a moment, as you spread the arms to the sides, palm facing upwards and out-stretched near ear level. Feel the life force rising from the throat up the head to the crown center, and spreading out from the top of the head and emanating all around you. Release the contraction at the perineum.

7. Begin exhalation, by lowering the shoulders and returning the hands to its position in front of the throat, feeling the life-force descending to the throat center. Contract the chest muscles, and lowering the hands to the heart center, as the *prana* descends. Complete the exhalation by contracting the abdomen, lowering the hands to the navel, as the *prana* descends to the navel center. At the end of the exhalation, the hands are resting on top of the thighs, as at the beginning of the cycle.

8. Repeat twice more and then completely relax.

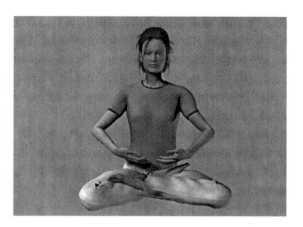

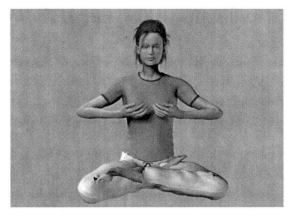

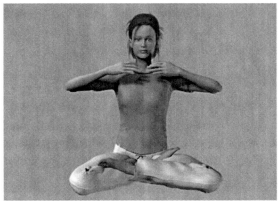

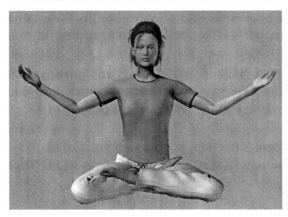

Figure 2: Prana Mudra

Enthusiasm and Energetic Will

The spiritual journey is often long, full of detours and huge potholes. Anyone who has attempted to setup a regular practice of spiritual discipline will soon realize the ebb and flow of energy and motivation for following through with the initial resolution.

When we first get initiated into a spiritual discipline we are usually full of enthusiasm and strong resolve to achieve the goal of Self-Realization. We feel ourselves ready for all the challenges that may come our way and protected from all obstructions that we may encounter. However, soon after we leave the initiation hall, reality sets in and we start to wonder how we are going to live up to our commitment to practice daily everything that has been taught.

As days become weeks and weeks become months, doubts set in and the initial burst of enthusiasm has all but disappeared and the practice may be overcome by lethargy or the demands of a busy life-style. Why does this happen and how can we prevent it from occurring?

First, we must understand that the spiritual path is not one which is a graph-like straight line moving upwards at forty-five degrees or some other inclination, but more like a series of plateaus punctuated by a sharp upward jump. It is during the plateau periods when no apparent progress is being made that the students becomes dejected and would often give up. The plateaus are periods of consolidation and actualization of our potential and their lengths are determined by the intensity of practice as well as the karmic tendencies of the students.

Secondly, we must realize that our preconceptions and expectations are deadly to keeping up the enthusiasm for the practice. No amount of progress can live up to our expectations which grossly exaggerate the speed and power of the results. It is important to give up our expectations and be content with whatever comes during the practice, whether positive or negative.

Thirdly, we need to understand that the first wave of enthusiasm is emotion driven based on the momentum of the initiation and the interaction between teacher and student, as well as momentum driven because of the spiritual energy that is transmitted during an initiation. However, emotions are like clouds that pass fairly quickly through the sky and cannot be relied on to maintain a steady and regular rhythm.

The solution is to generate proactively the enthusiasm that is based on energetic will. This means that we must use our will-power and energy to power the enthusiasm for the practice.

Setting up regular times for the practice and not letting anything interfere with it is of paramount importance in making spiritual progress. It is more effective to have a daily practice of 30 minutes than to have a haphazard practice that in a week might be 5 or 6 hours long but some days are completely empty. It is best not to let a day slip by without practice because there is a constant accumulation of karmic tendencies and they grow harder to destroy and burn away as they become consolidated over time.

One should meet regularly with spiritually like-minded people to help support the enthusiasm. This might mean re-arranging our schedule and giving higher priority to these spiritual meetings than to other obligations. This might mean driving a longer distance to attend the meeting. It might even entail offering to host such events in one's home!

One should keep up a steady study habit and continue to read inspiring books, not at the expense of practice, but as a complement to continuously generate the requisite enthusiasm. Completely giving up reading books because one has received initiation into a spiritual path can become a trap unless one is highly self-motivated.

One of the best ways to generate enthusiasm is to participate in spiritual chanting which is usually part of devotional practice. Whatever one's path, even if it is considered to be highly meditation-based, there is always a need to connect with the source of love and joy. Spiritual chanting helps to activate this connection which then can be willfully channeled into enthusiasm for one's regular discipline.

The key is to realize that enthusiasm is not a passive and unchanging ingredient in our lives and we need to actively use our energy and will to activate and grow it within our hearts if we are to successfully cross the ocean of suffering.

Prosperity And Success

O Divine Source of All, gift us Your blessings in our lives.
Struggling in the temporary delusion of separateness,
we work and worry for our daily physical necessities.
Let us remember You, the One in All and the All in One.

O Divine Source of All, gift us with success in our lives.
Caught in the illusory trap of fear and unworthiness,
we sabotage our own efforts with thoughts of failure.
Let us remember You, the loving Father and Mother.

O Divine Source of All, gift us with happiness in our lives.
Immersed in the deafening roar of sense gratification,
we search and grasp in our external world for satisfaction.
Let us remember You, the Bliss within our hearts.

O Divine Source of All, gift us with prosperity in our lives.
Chained by the karmic bonds of past thoughts, words and
deeds,
we drown in the ocean of suffering for lack of basic needs.
Let us remember You, the destroyer of our negativities.

O Divine Source of All, gift us with contentment in our lives.
Stuck on the wheel of desires for more that generate more
desires,
we bounce in pain between the emotions of loss and gain.
Let us remember You, Light that drives dark of ignorance
away.

Is Money A Hindrance On The Spiritual Path?

Money is a form of energy. It is earned by work or some other effort and is useful as a standard means of exchange. The mere possession of money or material wealth by itself is not counterproductive to spiritual progress. It is the attachment to or obsession with money that is a great hindrance. Wealth can be used for helping others and for maintaining a balanced lifestyle to enable one to follow the spiritual path without worries about food or shelter. However, if one spends most of one's time trying to get more and more wealth while neglecting one's practice, then there is little hope for that life. On the other hand, if one is so poor that one cannot support oneself or one's family, then there will be difficulty in maintaining a strong practice. Let common sense and the example of past masters guide us.

A rich young man wanted to follow the Master Jesus, but the Lord saw that the man's heart was too attached to his wealth and so He told him to give away all his riches if he wanted to be a disciple. It is not because wealth per se is bad, but the attachment.

An ancient Indian sage, Janaka was also a wealthy king with much land and a grand palace. He was once in the forest attending his Master's lecture, together with many others, when reports came that the capital city was on fire and that the palace and all his riches were in danger. Everyone starting sneaking away to attend to their possessions, and only Janaka was left. After the Master had given the highest teachings, He asked the king why he did not attend to his palace, Janaka responded that he had able servants who could take care of such material things and even if his material riches were lost, they were not important and may be regained, but the spiritual riches being given by the Master might not be available again for many lifetimes. Soon,

28

the servants came and reported that all the fires were merely illusions and had mysteriously disappeared and that the king's possessions and his subjects were all fine – it had been the Master's test for his students.

Exercise:

1. Write down how you feel about money. Do you have enough? Do you think it's a hindrance or a help on the spiritual path or does it matter at all?

2. What would you do differently if you won a lot of money in the lottery tomorrow?

3. How would you feel if you lost all your money tomorrow? What would you do?

The Danger of Aversion

Everyone has their likes and dislikes but we are seldom aware of how our dislikes are responsible for some of our problems in life. We are not even aware sometimes of the source of our dislikes and their strength catches us by surprise.

The spiritual student is constantly reminded about the dangers of desires and the attraction or attachment to subjects or objects of the senses because they will cause more links in the chains that bind us to the material world and prevent us from soaring into the spiritual dimensions. However, equally insidious but often overlooked are our dislikes – our aversions to subjects or objects of the senses.

Of course, all of us have our preferences – one may like chocolate ice-cream while another prefers strawberry flavor and both don't like vanilla. There is no harm in this. However, it is the reaction to our encountering what we don't like that determine whether there is an aversion problem. If one over-reacts to being served vanilla ice-cream by throwing it on the floor or even at the unknowing server, then it is a problem. Or, if one feels ill or literally throws up when presented with the vanilla ice-cream, then it is a problem.

We don't normally react to something as innocuous as vanilla ice-cream, but there are many other phobias and deep-seated reaction patterns that can throw us of our stride. Common aversions include the taste or sight of certain vegetables, to being on time, to certain colors, to certain insects or animals and even to certain people. Another common aversion is the avoidance of self-analysis.

The genesis of aversion is the avoidance of pain. This serves a useful feedback mechanism – we should all have an aversion to putting our hands into a burning fire. Those of us with vivid imaginations can already see the crisping skin, smell the burning flesh, and hear the scream of pain. What about a painful relationship? It becomes a reaction pattern to have a gut-wrenching spasm at the sight of someone whom one has broken off from.

Aside from the natural reactions to real dangers, physical, emotional or mental, we have also built up imaginary avoidance reactions. The child who refuses to eat certain foods out of pique eventually builds up an aversion for them. More seriously, the person with an eating disorder can form an aversion to all foods.

The development of equanimity is the key to being free from attraction or aversion. One should develop a steady mental attitude towards all events, rather then be subject to the rollercoaster of likes and dislikes. Long periods of meditation and spiritual practice are needed to accomplish a state of equanimity. This can be speeded up by the practice of forgiveness and love for those whom we have formed negative reaction patterns. For objects of avoidance, one can visualize their enjoyment and slowly erode the negative mental patterns and form new ones of tolerable non-preference.

It is just as necessary to de-program our aversions as it is to de-program ourselves from our obsessions. Whether it is avoiding certain people, food, movies or television programs, books, music etc., one should become aware of our "peculiarities" and seek to overcome them consciously. One can only be free when one is free from such reaction patterns.

Focus on Asanas –
Bow Pose (Dhanurasana)

The bow pose is one of the primary postures because it stimulates the navel center and energizes the whole body, strengthening the digestive system and promoting mental self-control. Therapeutically, it is beneficial for preventing diabetes and treating gastrointestinal disorders, menstrual disorders and obesity.

Anyone with high-blood pressure, heart disease, colitis, peptic or duodenal ulcers should avoid this posture.

Basic Technique: Lie down on your front with forehead on the floor, arms by the side and feet slightly apart. Fold the knees and bring the feet towards the buttocks. Stretch your hands back and hold on to the feet. Exhale completely and lift both knees and chest up simultaneously. Raise thighs and chest more by extending the feet towards the ceiling and the head as far back as possible. Maintain the pose for about one minute and breathe normally. Exhale and return to resting position.

Refer figure 3 for illustrations on the bow pose.

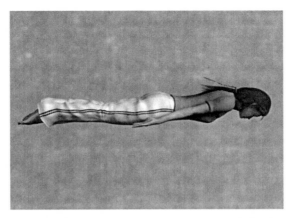

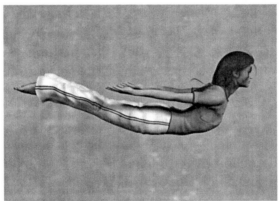

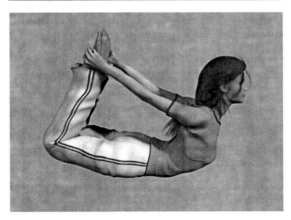

Figure 3: Bow Pose

Remembrance

In our hearts we all know that if we can remember our mistakes, we will eventually learn not to repeat them.

At every phase of our lives, we are often subjected to learning experiences from which we are expected to form our own conclusions and make the best of every situation. However, it is a very ad-hoc and haphazard process without definite rules and highly dependent on inherited like/dislikes, family and cultural programming.

During our childhood, we learn about the world around us and about the capabilities of our bodies. We find that putting our hands into the flames of a fire will hurt and that it is true even if we repeat the experience – eventually, we learn to avoid flames.

We learn to deal with relationships during our teenage years – what works and what doesn't work. Friendship or loneliness results from our choices and actions. There are no rules – what works for one person may not work for another.

We learn about responsibilities during our adult phase – supporting ourselves and forming new family units. During old age, we begin to learn the futility of all our hopes and desires and adjust ourselves for the coming death experience.

There is a great virtue known as *smriti* which is the **remembrance of our experiences** so that we **take actions that produce positive results** and **avoid actions that produce negative results**.

Unfortunately for us, we forget our life lessons and even when we do sort of remember, we choose to ignore them.

We sometimes would overindulge in food or drink even though

we know that we will suffer the consequences. The drunk who suffers the hangover will start drinking again after a few days. The drunken driver knows that there are serious consequences both to oneself and to others but continue a dangerous course of action. Obesity is the result of people ignoring the experience of ever-eating. Why are smokers unable to quit their life-threatening habit?

Remembrance is not only the development of memory but also the development of will-power. It is often the case that we subconsciously try to forget our experiences so that we do not have to make the difficult decisions.

The first step in recovery is to examine one's life and record the areas where one seems to be constantly having problems whether in one's health, one's professional life, one's relationships or one's lack of happiness. There is usually no difficulty in identifying the problem areas. For instance, if one consistently enters into troubled relationships with certain types of people, it is evident that there is some life lesson which needs to be resolved.

The second step is to acknowledge the specific area which needs remembrance. Acknowledgement is a mental acceptance of the issue at hand. If one refuses to accept a problem then it negates the possibility of taking personal responsibility and action.

The third step is to set aside time – I recommend at least fifteen minutes three times a day – in the morning, during the lunch hour and just before retiring for the night. During these three periods of time, one should recollect the issue, acknowledge it and willfully apply oneself to resolving it by remembering to avoid the causal factors in the present.

There are those who wonder why we cannot remember the lessons that we have learned or failed to learn in previous lives, but do not even make the effort to remember the lessons from the present life.

There is an ancient prayer that says, "O, Divine, please help me to remember!" Let us learn from our experiences now.

Exercise:

1. Write down an area in your life that you can identify as having a recurring problem:

2. Write down the mistakes that you think you are making that cause you to have the problem:

3. Write down the solutions to the mistakes - things you can do to prevent the mistakes from happening:

Once or twice everyday at a set time, read and remember what you have written down.

Should A Spiritual Aspirant Rely On Astrology?

Let us be very clear upfront - a spiritual aspirant should only rely on his or her own efforts to practice the discipline given by the spiritual guide on the path. There is no substitute for one's own regular practice.

Astrology, especially the Indian form called *Jyotish*, is the artful science which attempts to glean the secrets of the planetary mapping of each person's life potential and probable life trajectory. This is similar to the current science that is making progress in mapping one's genetic code – this can give indications of susceptibility to certain diseases before they can occur, as well as certain emotional and mental tendencies due to hormonal and chemical imbalances. The genetic code is in the microscopic level while the planetary code is in macroscopic level.

The problems with astrology is that it has become mystified over time and burdened with dubious accretions that have no basis in reality. There was a proliferation of dubious practitioners who caused this ancient science to fall into disrepute. Of course, there are very sincere and knowledgeable practitioners even now, but it is difficult to ascertain those who are true *jyotishis* from those who are opportunists.

Those who live a materialistic life are more prone to behave predictably according to their innate tendencies or karma, while those who have decided to swim upstream by pursuing the spiritual goal of self-realization are less subject to their *karmic* tendencies. The consequence is that a Self-Realized *yogi* is no longer subject to *karma* and therefore cannot be predictable under any form of fortune telling.

For spiritual seekers on the path any method that claim to have predictive capabilities may be helpful if it can provide information about health – such as tendencies towards particular sicknesses, so that preventive measures such as a proper dietary and exercise plan may be implemented.

My personal favorite use for *jyotish* is to help seekers with useful information on the path, such as present life-lessons, past life *karma*, correct life-path, best choice of *mantra*, or identification of *Ishtadeva* (personal form of liberation).

Sometimes, there are advanced people who seem to be using methods such as astrology, palmistry, dice or cards, but may be actually accessing their intuition or higher faculties to make predictions rather than the rules of the method. Such psychic talents should not be over-utilized or relied on due to the strain they may put on the psychic sooner or later. Only realized *yogis* have the unlimited access to these psychic sources but they will seldom need to use them.

I discourage any kind of future forecasting with any kind of "fortune-telling" method primarily because they will seldom be accurate. Most "predictions" are either so general that they can fit multiple scenarios or are self-fulfilling prophecies, made true, by the highly suggestive. Even the best of forecasts are only one of many possible event trajectories that can be altered by one's choices – of course, the astrologer will choose the most probable trend by observing the current state and deducing the likely course based on the *karmic* pattern.

It is best to cultivate the correct course of actions through the practice of the *yamas* and *niyamas* and surrendering oneself to the Divine. Let our *karma* work itself out rather than try to avoid it. It is sometimes possible to mitigate the *karmic* effects by the proper application of gemstones, *mantras* or other self-efforts such as pilgrimages, but this should be under the advice of a spiritual guide.

Nothing is fixed and unchangeable – the universe is very

dynamic and can be influenced by our choices. Only if we are too lazy or set in our ways, will we be following the flow of our *karmic* habits. It is different from the flow that happens when one truly surrenders to the Divine and events are then guided by the Divine Will. Do not confuse the two.

Celebrate Guru Purnima

Once a year, a day is set aside to commemorate one's teachers, especially one's spiritual mentors. This is the day called Guru Purnima and this year, it falls on Thursday, July 17th / Friday, July 18th.

Just as we honor our parents on Mother's Day and Father's Day, we honor those who have been responsible for our spiritual re-birth on this full-moon day of the seventh month.

The light of the Divine is within each and every one of us. However, it is hidden by the clouds of our ignorance and desires. A Spiritual Teacher or Master is one who can awaken the hidden light of divine knowledge within the seeker student.

Over time, more and more elaborate ceremonies have been created to celebrate the person and work of the spiritual mentor during this special day. It is not necessary to be conversant with these devotional rites in order to pay our respects. Of course, it is a great blessing if one has the opportunity to thank the Master in person. More often, we are separated by time and space from the Guru.

Whether one's Teacher is alive or working in higher planes, whether one is participating in a group or by oneself, it is only necessary to either have an image or a good visualization. Light a candle flame and a stick of incense. A good time to do this is around 6:30 pm to 7:00 pm. The seeker / student /disciple should offer a flower and fruit to the image of the Master with thanks and invite blessings for the coming year. If we have been taught any Guru stotras/mantras including the Hanuman Chalisa, this would be a good time to say them aloud. The most important part of the "ceremony" is to practice the spiritual discipline given by the Master – this is the greatest thanks you can give to any Teacher!

In case one feels doubtful that the grace of the Master has appeared in one's life and is till in the searching mode, this is a good time to ask for the manifestation of the spiritual guide in one's life. Place an image of the Master of the Master of all Masters, Lord Shiva and offer the fruit and flowers to Him, chanting 'Om Nama Shivaya' and if you know it, the Karpoora Aarti. It is said that when the student is ready, the Master will appear – one needs to be ever on the lookout and be prepared. Tune in to your soul-heart and seek there for the ever-present inspirational guidance.

This day is also an opportunity for each of us to re-examine our progress on the spiritual path, to re-affirm our commitment to our practice and to re-connect with the spiritual guide within. Traditionally, on this day, our connection with our inner guide is the strongest and the veil of illusion thinnest, and therefore, we should make our sincere effort to tune into and receive the grace of our True Self.

For those who are Teachers and spiritual guides, it is a day to selflessly transmit the blessings and grace of the Divine to all the seekers that are in your stream of consciousness – to pour forth your soul force to those struggling in the mire of Maya. It is an opportunity to grow further in one's quest to be a better Servant of Humanity, to be more capable to serve all who are drawn to you.

JAI GURU – We bow to the Divine Teacher within all of us!

Mantra Yoga

One of the great paths of liberation is by the practice of mantras or spiritually charged sonic patterns formed from the Sanskrit language.

The word *mantram* combines the root *manas* (mind) with *tram* (protection) so the literal meaning is mind-protection. The mind is subject to innumerable perturbations that constantly disturb and keep it from the stillness that can lead the soul to higher consciousness. The proper practice of a mantra will lead the soul to the realization of the Self.

Since the effectiveness of mantras depend on their vibrations, their correct pronunciation become very important. They can be practiced by chanting aloud or by repeating mentally – some of them are meant to be mentally repeated for the purpose of being internalized, while others give emphasis to external effects. Mantras have been known to promote self-healing, spiritual development, as well as beneficial effects on the world around us.

Mantras can be used as the only means of spiritual liberation or as part of an integrated yogic system. Most yogic paths utilize some form of mantra or another in their techniques.

The most basic mantra is Om which is known as the "pranava mantra," the source of all mantras. It is the humming sound of creation because it is the vibration of the universe and the sound uttered by the Divine Creatrix. More complex sound patterns utilize the sound of Om in their beginning. It is used as an address for the Divine.

Om is the principal mantra given by Patanjali in his Yoga Sutras. It can be chanted aloud, whispered or repeated mentally. In higher yogic techniques, instead of repeating the sound, the student should listen and try to hear the sound within and without

– forming a powerful connection with the Universal Soul.

Nowadays, the emphasis is on the mantras which utilize bija or seed sounds because of their easier pronunciation, and prevalent use in tantric systems. Mantras were originally conceived in the ancient scriptures known as the Vedas. When they are crafted into two-line verses, they are called "shlokas."

The following is from Rigveda X-191-4:

> *Samaani va aakutih*
> *samaanaa hrdayaani vah.*
> *Samaanamastu vo mano*
> *yathaa vah susahaasati.*

> Let us unite our intentions.
> May your hearts also be in unison.
> United be the thoughts of all,
> That we may all happily agree.

The repetition of this mantra tends to promote a team consciousness and help a group to achieve common goals. It is very helpful to chant in a group.

Focus On - Mantra

There are *mantras* which should be repeated aloud in order to have the desired effects on the external world, that is, the environment and physical body. There are also mantras which should be repeated mentally only, in order to internalize their effects for wholly spiritual purposes.

There are also some mantras which can be practiced both aloud and mentally. In general, we can repeat these powerful vibrations first, aloud, then in a whisper and finally mentally. These three modes of repetition give powerfully enhanced effects on the physical, energetic/emotional, and mental/causal complex of human beings.

The following is one *mantra* which has been repeated everyday by spiritual seekers for thousands of years and is one I recommend to chant before your daily practice:

Om
Asatoma Sadgamaya
Tamasoma Jyotirgamaya
Mrityorma Amritamgamaya.

O, Divine
Lead me away from untruth to Truth
Lead me away from darkness to Light
Lead me away from death to Immortality.

Repeat it three times aloud, three times in a whisper, and three times silently. The best time is before meditation in the morning.

This mantra sums up simply and powerfully the aspiration of all spiritual seekers as well as the process that leads one to enlightenment.

Proper Use Of A Mala For Mantra Practice

One of the oldest and extremely effective spiritual paths is that of Mantra Yoga. The key is the initiation into an appropriate power or meditation sound pattern called a mantra by a teacher capable of transmitting the mantra to someone else.

Whether you have been initiated into a mantra practice or enjoying some mantra from an audio CD or even a book, if you are serious about practicing, you would need to use a mala or a rosary of one hundred and eight beads. The mala is used for counting the number of repetitions of the specific mantra. A practice generally requires the repetition of 108 counts or a multiple of 108 per session, with an ultimate goal of reaching a certain number such as 108,000 or 144,000 or even 1,080,000.

Since the mala is such an important tool in mantra practice, over the generations a large body of mystique has arisen over its proper use. A lot of the lore may be questionable, but much is quite symbolic as well as practical.

To understand some of the guidelines, it is necessary keep in mind that it is basic to the mystique of the mala that the beads retain some of the power and energy from the mantra itself. This means that the mala becomes a storage medium for mantric power and energy – this is especially true for one made from the rudraksha beads.

There are some practitioners who actually hide their malas under a bag as they count out the repetitions so as to prevent others from "stealing" their energy. This is somewhat extreme and most practitioners need not worry about such an event occurring.

I would recommend the following cautionary guidelines:

1. Use a bag to hold your mala rather than just putting it into your pockets as it will easily get damaged from frequent taking in and out or even get inadvertently lost.
2. Do not wear the mala that you are using for mantra practice as your body will then re-absorb the energy. If one wishes to wear a mala, it should be a separate one used only for wearing.
3. Never drop the mala on the floor or let someone else handle it as that will drain the energy.
4. Hold the mala with your second and third /ring fingers and do not touch it with the first finger as it is considered to have egoistic energy.
5. When you finish one round of 108 and wish to continue another round, do not go over the head bead which is not counted – one should flip the mala over and go back the way you had come.
6. If you are practicing more than one mantra, it is better to use a separate mala for the second mantra – best not to mix mantras on one mala.
7. If your mala gets broken and the beads are separated, do not try to mend it, but retire it away in a bag under you alter. A broken mala can no longer hold the energy and also may have a negative effect on your mantric practice.
8. The left hand is not used for mantric practice.
9. If you cannot complete the mala at some session, you can use a pin or clip to mark the location where you stopped, and continue from there when you have time – you do not need to start all over again.
10. Only a rudrasksha mala can be used for Shiva mantras or Shakti mantras – do not use crystal or lotus or some other material.

Try to get the best quality mala that you can as a low quality one will easily break during you practice. Smaller beads are used for mantra practice while malas with large beads are only used for wearing.

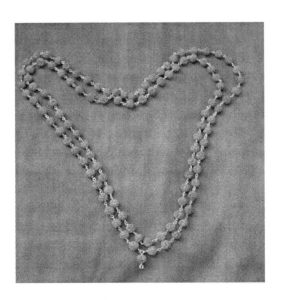

Figure 4: quality rudrakshamala

Samadhi-Prajna

Those who are aspiring to achieve super-conscious states of blissful unity called samadhi must first develop samadhi-prajna or discriminative wisdom. This is not the wisdom that arises during or after reaching super-consciousness, but rather that wisdom which is a pre-requisite.

This is important to understand because there are those who believe that one can attain samadhi states without first developing and displaying this wisdom in thought, word and deed. Indeed there are those who even claim to have experienced samadhi and do not display the post-samadhi wisdom that is a mark of those who have achieved a stabilized super-conscious state. We will examine the post-samadhi wisdom in a future article, and confine ourselves to the pre-samadhi wisdom today.

During the course of a sincere spiritual practice, flashes of insight occur. These insights happen when the higher mind, the buddhi is able to bypass the oversight of the ego (ahamkara) and the sense muddling of the lower mind (manas). Normal knowledge is based on the lower mind which operates with the five sensory inputs as well as the logical operation of inference. Insight occurs with direct knowing and without the five senses or logical inference. Insight is necessary because reality is beyond the five senses or the logical operation of the lower mind.

As one's practice matures and progresses, these flashes of insight become more and more frequent until they become continuous and the seeker is always in tune with the higher mind. As the insight mindfulness stabilizes, it is transformed into the pre-samadhi wisdom. In this state, one is able to discriminate between right and wrong in every moment and is able to make informed choices that obviously have karmic repercussions.

It is the continuous flow of pre-samadhi wisdom which is characteristic of those who have reached higher states of consciousness on the brink of super-consciousness unity bliss. There is also a bliss in the pre-samadhi wisdom which shadows that of samadhi bliss because of the continuous flow and connection with the higher mind.

The laws of reality are no longer a mystery to those who have attained to the pre-samadhi wisdom. However, they have not yet penetrated into that which underlie the laws of reality – for that, they must wait for the post-samadhi wisdom.

The attainment of pre-samadhi wisdom is a long and arduous process of removing the layers of illusion wrought by the sensory lower mind and the trickster ego. However, one should not confuse this lower attainment with that of the true samadhi state, nor should one enjoy it to the detriment of the final goal of Self-Realization.

I'm often asked why I don't describe this or other states of consciousness in even more detail and my answer is always that one should only know enough to be helpful to the path and not so much that it becomes a hindrance. The Masters of the past have time and time again observed that human beings have a great capacity for self-delusion and the powerful team of the lower mind and ego can derail sincere students into believing they have experiences which are only mental dreams or visions that are not the real attainment of higher consciousness. It is like an actor playing superman who believes that he is actually superman – hopefully he will not try to jump out of a window. The mind is capable of recreating all sorts of pseudo-experiences that will delude someone to make claims far beyond their actual attainment.

Olympics and Self-Realization

Every four years, a large part of the world takes time out of their busy lives to cheer on the athletes that have made it into the Olympic Games. A week ago, I watched the spectacle of the opening ceremony in Beijing, China and it was indeed awe-inspiring. The beauty and scale of the pageant made much ado about harmony and the welcome of friendship – such laudable emotions are indeed inspiring and something to aspire towards.

However, just a few hours later, the representatives who mingled easily together the previous night, were literally and figuratively at each others' throats. They all had the same goal – to win a gold medal at all costs. Most of them have trained hard all their lives and dedicated every waking moment to their dreams of the elusive golden icon. It makes for gripping entertainment and we all cheer on our favorites, applauding the ones who succeed and shaking our heads at the failed and fallen heroes. This is the way of competition – one winner and many losers.

Please realize that unlike an Olympic event in which there is only one gold medal winner, Self-Realization has unlimited number of gold medals!

It is unfortunate that many spiritual seekers and otherwise sincere yogic practitioners behave as if the realization of the true Self and achievement of our highest potential is a competitive race. Students within the same group vie for the attention of their spiritual guide and compete to show off their achievements rather than serve in the spirit of selflessness that is necessary for spiritual attainment. The intensification of the ego is counterproductive to the practice of Yoga.

There is no attainment for those who compete on how well they can hold a physical posture or how long they can hold their breath or how long they can hold their meditation without moving, only pain and suffering. Practice has to be performed for practice sake without attachment or desire in order to reach higher consciousness and any competitiveness with others or even with oneself serves to strengthen the ego.

There are some spiritual guides who encourage competitiveness by their students as a way to spur them on the path. However, this is two-edged sword and eventually the ego of short-term achievements will be a barrier to Self-Realization and we can only hope that the teacher is there to knock down the inflated ego eventually.

Jealousy of fellow spiritual students is another barrier to higher awareness. It is often observed that when one student seems to make tremendous progress, others seek to tear down the one who has apparently moved ahead. This is a symptom of our cultural upbringing which has an underlying presumption that someone making progress in any field does so at the cost of others, that life is a zero-sum game – if someone wins, someone else must lose. This is not the case on the spiritual path – there can be as many winners as there are spiritual aspirants. We must re-program our basic assumptions and remove the subconscious blocks that have been built up without our understanding so that we can rejoice and applaud the progress of our fellow seekers.

If one person achieves Self-Realization, everyone on earth benefits from that one's efforts. Objectively, the realized person can help others on the path. Subjectively, we all share the same divine essence – we are One in the Divine and so share in some part the achievement, but for the intercession of the individuating ego.

Just as in the Olympics, teams compete against each other and sometimes resort to name calling and badgering to win some minute advantage on the field of battle, so also do so-called spiritual organizations denounce each other or claim some superior legitimacy.

The rhetoric endorsed by some organizations confine themselves to coming up with buzzwords that confuse the sincere seekers, with the intention to ensnare them into their fold with promises of quick and effortless redemption, liberation or bliss-full experiences. There is a game of one-upmanship in the marketing and advertising campaigns, just as there is between rival companies or countries or teams. The distinctive character of a spiritual goal is put aside for the sake of expediency and growth – the metric for material success is transferred to the spiritual world.

The truth is that spiritual groups and organizations can only help the sincere practitioner on the path – they are not substitutes for one's daily meditation. Devotion to any organization cannot lead to salvation, only devotion to the Divine.

Seek out those groups and organizations that offer sincere help without requiring mindless obedience to their rules or strictures against belonging to another group. The spectacular failures of religious organizations should be a warning to spiritual groups to eschew such retrogressions. Yoga is not a religion.

There is no competition within the Divine Consciousness, only within our limited minds. Let us free ourselves from such limitations and embrace our true nature of one-ness. Let us free ourselves from competitiveness and jealousies and open ourselves to the infinities, to the unlimited number of gold medals available beyond the Olympia of minor gods and athletes of physical excellence. Let us extend our hands of friendship to all the fellow travelers on the path.

Focus on:
Affirmations

An affirmation is a positive thought or statement that you repeat to yourself and implant in your inner consciousness as a source of inspiration for your present and future actions. Once secured in your subconscious mind, it guides your thoughts and actions in a chosen direction. You can use the power of affirmations to overcome certain undesirable traits and negative and habitual thought patterns in your mind or deal with some weakness in your personality affirmatively.

Using positive affirmations you can instruct your body and mind to act in a certain way. You can overcome the barriers that stand in between you and your true Self. You can send subtle thought forces into your consciousness and powerfully alter your thinking and behavior. Using positive affirmations, you can heal yourself in astonishing ways. You can stay motivated and focused on your path to spiritual enlightenment. You can truly transform your personality and make yourself more acceptable and at peace with yourself, overcoming many problems in your life, problems that exist because of some inherent deficiency or debility with your attitude, behavior or thinking, as a result of your *karmic* load.

Positive affirmations may not get you every thing you want in your life, but they can help you establish an environment in which you have greater opportunities to shape your life and alter the course of your actions. They can help you overcome the feelings of frustration and helplessness and make you feel confident, self-reliant and responsible for your actions and thoughts. You can face the challenges of your life more confidently and with the conviction that you're not a mere pawn in the hands of some unknown fate. You can practically do anything that's humanly possible and within the field of your reality. It is possible to use affirmations for goals which are not particularly spiritually oriented, but such changes in life direction are generally band-aids which do not address the fundamental issues, which are generally *karmic* and spiritual, and therefore it is advisable to put more of your energy to solving these ultimate problems.

The characteristics of successful affirmations:

Following are some of the suggestions on how to make your affirmation work for you and bring success and happiness in your daily life:

- The affirmation should be appropriate to the problem that you want to deal with.

- Use words that focus on the end result desired.

- Repeat the affirmation regularly until it is firmly integrated with your consciousness and become part of your natural response to the intended problem.

- Associate your affirmation consciously and persistently with the problem you want to resolve.

- Balance your negative thought or fear with the positive affirmation

- Write the affirmation down on a paper or some book and keep it within easy reach.

- Memorize the affirmation for easy repetition.

- Start your day with positive affirmations and remember them before you go to bed. During the day, use them on as many occasions as you can, and definitely when you need them most - when there is a need to reinforce a desired behavior or state of mind or counter a problem or situation you are facing.

- Keep your affirmation simple, using action words that invoke positive imagery and appeal to your mind and sense directly.

- Make your affirmations personal and in first person. Feel the need for them strongly. Experience the sense of responsibility as you think of them.

- Use positive words only. Avoid negative expressions. Say, "I'm achieving this state of mind or reality," instead of "I don't want to be like this or that or I don't want to do this or that."

- Act as if your affirmations are already working and yielding positive results. Express your gratitude to the Divine.

- Add the power of visualization to the force of your affirmations. Visualize how your affirmations can change your life and your personality.

- Use the power of *Yoga Nidra* to create the environment for the most effective seeding of the affirmation on the receptive consciousness.

There can be many appropriate uses of affirmations to counteract our karmic limitations and predispositions. For those who are unsure what to use, I always recommend affirmations that work on the five yamas – these are the five self-restraints that are recommended by Sage Patanjali in his treatise on Yoga – ahimsa (non-violence), satya (truth), asteya (non-stealing), brahmacharya (reversal of energy inwards) and aparigraha (non-attachment.)

It is difficult for most of us to practice *ahimsa* or nonviolence in thought, word or deed, since we are prone to anger and fear, which requires the antidote of love. The same situation exists for the other four restraints.

An example of an affirmations is as follows:

I am completely filled with Divine Love and I express love to all beings under all circumstances.

Exercise: Think of three virtues that you wish to increase in yourself and try to write down one affirmation for each of these positive traits in your own words.

The Threat of Mortality

Last week I read about an experiment that was going to be performed along the France-Swiss border. This physics experiment involved the Hadron Collider, a twenty-seven kilometer underground tunnel that cost $10B and many years of collaboration from hundreds of scientists. The goal is apparently to learn more about the origins of the universe by colliding elementary particles together. What was even more interesting to the ordinary person was the hopefully tongue-in-cheek observation that there was a possibility that the experiment would produce a black hole that would swallow up the earth. Would we wake up the next day or be extinguished in our sleep?

The world gets a rude awakening every now and then – a threat of a colliding asteroid or a nuclear war that would destroy all life. What would you do if you knew the world was going to end tomorrow?

Would you rush to satisfy as many of your desires as possible or would you run to your religious church or temple to find solace? Would you find your best friend or try to seek your own divine nature by continuing your spiritual practice?

When we are young we live our lives as if we will live forever. Immersed in our own trivial personal concerns we usually give no thought to death. But as one grows older and mortality asserts itself, one becomes more and more aware of the fleeting nature of life.

It takes some unusual occurrence, some sudden shock to wake us up from our slumber of mediocrity. Humanity has had the capability to destroy itself for the last fifty years but have managed to put that stress into the background and consciously ignore the threat. Only when there is fear of an imminent disaster do we take stock of ourselves and are forced to re-examine our lives.

In a recent movie, an old man facing his sudden mortality writes up a list of everything he would like to do before his death – he called it his "bucket list." Such is the reaction of many people, even when faced with imminent termination - the satisfaction of desires is uppermost in their minds. It is because of these unsatisfied desires that the soul is reborn again and again. Intellectually, we know this, but the force of these desires is beyond our control. Can we ever satisfy all our desires – the hydra-headed monster that grows ten new heads every time we cut off one?

We do not know when our life will end but need to live as if every day is our last and make the best use of our time to reach our goal of Self-Realization. Should we wait for some death threat before we look towards our own true nature? When one starts to dig for water only when dying of thirst, the chance of success is slim.

This reminds me of the inspiring example of a great saint called Ramana Maharshi. As a boy, he was suddenly assailed by a great fear of death and this forced him to examine his true nature. He spontaneously began to penetrate beyond the identification of body and mind. He reached a super-consciousness state by meditating on "who am I?" Although he was illiterate and had not learned any meditation techniques, due to his past life yogic practices and the stimulus of a death threat, he realized his innate immortality. This is very unusual and almost impossible for us.

Death serves a very important function – without it, we would continue on our path of sense compulsion. It was the sight of death that finally moved Prince Siddhartha to become the Buddha.

Life is precious and uncertain. All the sages have counseled that we make the best use of our limited stay on earth and follow the path of Self-Realization. Even if we do not achieve our true nature in one life, we will surely do so in the next.

Exercise:

1. Write down what you would do if you knew that you are going to die tomorrow. List out what you can do within twenty-four hours.

2. Review the list and write down beside each action whether it is for satisfying a desire, helping someone or something for attaining higher consciousness.

3. Write down how you feel about the activities after reviewing them against the three criteria.

4. Now prioritize the activities.

5. Do your priorities lead you to do something different with your life right now?

The Source of Prosperity

In Ancient India, there was a rich and powerful king who was never satisfied with his lands and wealth. He was especially jealous of his cousins, whom he'd plotted against many times. The eldest cousin was an upright and noble king, who always managed to re-gain his prosperity, despite all the subterfuges.

The jealous king went to his aged and blind father to learn from him the explanation on how the noble king always came out on top. The father instructed his son by telling him the following story:

There were incessant wars between the forces of light, led by the hero-god Indra and the forces of darkness led by various demon kings. At one time, the demon king was Prahlada, who had transformed his nature to such an extent that he was able to annex the domains of the gods and men by the force of his character and made himself Lord of the three worlds.

Dispossessed, but undaunted, Indra went to the high priest of the gods, Brihaspati, and with all humility, begged him to teach him the means by which he could re-gain his spiritual leadership. Brihaspati taught him the means and said that if he practiced steadfastly it would lead him eventually to paramount virtue.

Indra then asked how that path leading him to spiritual and moral character could be shortened, and Brihaspati counseled him to go learn from the teacher of all the demons. However when the king of light approached the teacher of all the demons, he was in turn counseled to learn directly from his nemesis Prahlada.

Putting on the guise of a spiritual seeker, Indra approached Prahlada and begged him to teach him the path to prosperity. However Prahlada was fully occupied with the administration all the three worlds and told the disguised Indra that he had no time to take a student. In response Indra fell down at the feet of Prahlada and pleaded that he would wait as long as necessary for instruction from such a supreme preceptor.

Pleased with such earnestness, Prahlada chose an auspicious hour to begin and proceeded to teach the highest wisdom to his student, the hero-god. After receiving the teaching in reverence and humility, Indra inquired of Prahlada how he had obtained lordship of the three worlds.

Prahlada replied, "I am never proud that I am king; I do not treat the learned and holy ones with derision. Listening to their words of wisdom I discipline myself and give liberally. They speak to me in confidence and I let myself be guided by them in all things. The sages establish me safely and securely in *dharma* as the bees confine honey in the honeycomb. I have conquered anger and my senses are under my control. In this way I live in the company of those whose speech keep pace with their understanding, delighting in the light of knowledge. The words of wisdom coming from the lips of a learned person – that is the basis of all prosperity."

After some time had passed, pleased with his student's service and attention, Prahlada offered him a boon and asked him to request whatever he wanted. Whereupon Indra said, "if you are pleased with me and would give me anything I ask for, I would ask for the gift of your character. Please give me your moral character."

Naturally, Prahlada was taken aback by this request and was quite beside himself for a while. Yet a promise is a promise and a boon granted could not be revoked by a noble person. He therefore regretfully made a gift of his entire moral character to the disguised Indra who immediately thanked him and left.

Prahlada was sitting and thinking about what had happened when a spirit of great luster emanated from his body and in response to his startled question said, "I am your moral character and you have divested yourself of me and so I'm going to reside in your student." It then disappeared into the body of Indra.

No sooner had this spirit disappeared, and another great light arose from Prahlada and said, "I am *dharma* and I'm going to your student because I can only reside where there is moral character. Then a third spirit came out of Prahlada's body, even brighter than the previous two and declared himself to be the spirit of truth or *satya* who goes where *dharma* goes.

Immediately after the departure of *satya*, the spirit of good conduct *vritta* rose up together with the spirit of strength, and both left, because strength and good conduct are inseparable.

To make matters worse, a lustrous woman of great divinity appeared and prepared to leave. Prahlada tried to stop her, but she responded, "I am Lakshmi - everything that makes for whatever it is auspicious and for prosperity, and I must follow the strength and valor which has left you."

Prahlada realized how his pride and rashness had deprived him of his high moral character. This humbled him and he completely surrendered himself to the Absolute Divine, from whom he had received everything, and to whom he had been so devoted in his childhood. He gave up all desires for the material world and achieved liberation.

So this is how the Lord of the gods, Indra recovered lordship of the three worlds, by learning the secret of moral character from Prahlada. This secret is, "in thought, word and deed, one should refrain from harming any creature. Compassion and giving are the marks of good character. One should not do what may injure another or whatever one would feel ashamed of. Do only that which evokes approval in the assembly of sages. This is the sum and essence of moral character. Even though some people may appear to be prosperous in the world who are not strong in moral character, their prosperity will not last long for its roots are neither deep nor strong. Therefore acquire the virtue of moral character if you wish to attain to lasting prosperity."

Unfortunately, the jealous king did not listen to his father and left unsatisfied. Soon after, he forced a great war against his cousins, but even though he had much larger forces, he was totally destroyed by the upright king.

Prosperity and Success are dependent on strength and valor, which in turn are dependent on truth and right action, which in turn are dependent on virtue.

The First Breath

When a baby is born from the womb and takes its first breath, the cycle of life begins. This first breath is part and parcel of the traumatic birth experience that serves to spread the baby's awareness outwards towards the external world.

While in the relative safety of the mother's womb, the senses were limited to their immediate environment which is kept fairly consistent and buffered from larger variations. At birth, the baby is subjected to an overload in all of its senses – the loud noises, the rough touch on the skin, the images impinging on the open eyes, the tastes from the open mouth and the weird smells. During the baby's subsequent development, all the mental power is spent on trying to accommodate the sense impressions and interact with the external environment.

Yogis in deep meditation have been able to see how the life-force or prana is dispersed from its core center to the periphery of the senses with the first breath. This outward movement of the prana becomes established as the automatic human reaction of entrapment in the five senses.

The irony is that when we start to pursue a spiritual path, we need to learn how to reverse this habitual outward flow of the prana. We need to redirect the pranic flow inwards and this is known as the yogic process of pratyahara or sense-withdrawal. In order to be able to reverse the flow of the prana, we need first to learn its control by the practice of pranayama or breath control. Without developing pranayama, it would be difficult to enter into pratyahara.

The yogis in their super-conscious states become aware that on the average, a human being would take 21,060 breaths every twenty-four hours and further that our life-span is mostly determined at birth with the first breath. This is because the amount of birth prana can only sustain a certain number of breaths before running out. Some of us are born with greater amounts of birth prana and so have a longer life-span barring other karmic factors. The total number of one's allocated breaths at birth determines the maximum number of our days.

One of the many reasons yogis recommend slower and deeper breathing is that it would lead to longer life spans!

A spiritual practice highly prized by spiritual teachers is that of japa. This is the constant repetition of one of the names of the Divine. What is not widely known is that real japa happens when the Name is repeated in conjunction with the breath. Something magical happens when one is able to co-ordinate every breath with the Name – the prana is redirected and pulled inwards towards its original center, away from the five senses. This is essential to reversing the effect of the first breath.

When one can maintain japa for 21,060 breaths, the prana becomes stabilized internally and the mind is established in high states of concentration that can lead to ecstatic states of unity consciousness or samadhi.

The true rebirth or second birth is the reversal of the outward direction of the first breath into an inward centric flow that can power the rocket ship of the soul towards the True Self.

Focus On Meditation: Physical Steadiness

In order to achieve success in concentration and subsequently to enter into meditative states, it is essential to be able to sit still without any movement for certain periods of time. This is due to the fact that when the body moves, the mind moves and concentration is broken. It is therefore important to give time for practicing a steady sitting posture.

Practice:
1. choose one of the recommended postures such as siddhasana, padmasana or vajrasana and then hold your spine erect. Adjust your head, neck and shoulders slightly back. Hands should be placed on the knees with chin or jnana mudra or with palms together. Close your eyes and focus on the breath for a few minutes.
2. Bring your awareness back to the body – focus on the position of the back, the arms and legs. Maintain this awareness for a minute or two.
3. Try to examine your body from the external perspective as if watching yourself while standing outside. Examine your body all around and from top to bottom.
4. Return to the body and feel it as a tree, with the legs rooted in the ground and the arms as branches of the tree. Feel yourself firmly attached to the ground and immobile.
5. Focus the mind on the physical sensations – any tension, itching or pain; any cold or heat – for a minute or two.
6. Become aware of the different parts of the body in sequential order – head, neck, shoulders, right arm, left arm, back, chest, abdomen, right leg, left leg, bottom and then the body as a whole. Perform this awareness three times.
7. Focus your mind on the concepts of steadiness and

immobility and give the command to the body to remain unmoving. Feel the body responding by becoming totally rigid. You will feel unable to move any part of the body without making a strong effort.

8. Become aware of the breath and gradually lose yourself in the incoming and outgoing breath as it gradually becomes more and more shallow and still. At this stage, concentration can begin.

9. To end the practice, return your attention to the body. Take a few long breaths and intone loudly Om three times.

Perseverance In Practice

The spiritual path is long an arduous and has many pitfalls and obstacles. We are often befuddled by our delusions and fall prey to illusions, thinking a true path is false or that we have achieved something when we have not.

Why does this happen? It is because of our karmic tendencies or samskaras operating in our field of experience including the very spiritual practices which are meant to burn them away. We cannot rely on our senses or our minds. We can only trust our heart and the spiritual guide. That is way it is useful to have a trusted guide on the path lest we fall by the wayside.

Once you've done your due diligence to select the guide and the path, the key to success is perseverance. Many have died and lived and died without achieving their true self because of doubts and the lack of intensity in their practice. Many have delayed their realization by prematurely giving up their daily practice. Do not join their ranks.

Practice, practice and practice more.

It is important to set your priorities – what do you want from this life? Something that you cannot take with you into the next life or something that can endure death? Besides one's karma, the only thing that survives death is spiritual practice. All the great sages have assured us that not one second of spiritual practice will be forgotten and that the fruits of our practice will last for eternity if need be.
You have nothing to lose and everything to gain or if you want to be very precise – you will lose everything and gain nothing, for only be giving up the impermanent things of life can you gain the immortality of the true Self which is nothing as it is not an object but you, Yourself.

It is perseverance that moves you to get up early in the morning from the warmth of your bed and complete your spiritual practice before going to work. It is perseverance that keeps your going even when everyone around you may be telling you that it's a waste of time and effort. It is perseverance that overcomes your despair, desperation, boredom, restlessness and doubt.

Set your sight on the priceless Divine and persevere in your practice, no matter the winds of emotional turmoil or the tsunami of physical and mental distress that come and go.

The Hero

We all like to watch movies or read a book about the heroic figure that battles against all odds and wins through by defeating formidable enemies. This can be the lone cowboy battling foes amidst the lonesome prairie or the space cadet fighting pirates in the starry void. It can be a person struggling through heavy bouts of debilitating depression or physical pain associated with chronic illnesses. These are all heroes.

However, it is striking and unique that in India, the heroic figure is most often the spiritual warrior, the one who conquers his inner nature to become liberated or enlightened. It is the one who seeks the truth of reality and who defeats all inner demons and achieves the true self. Such a one was Gautama, the Buddha and many others whose tales are still recounted to the children of this sacred land.

There is a story of another young boy named Nachiketa who provides a good example of somebody who really wanted to know and understand himself. Nachiketa's father was sage Vajashravasa, who once conducted a great ceremony, in which he offered all he had. He had used all he owned to buy cows, but because of his poverty, he could only afford lean and old cows. In order to honor his father, the boy bravely offered himself as part of the offering.

The little boy asked, "Father, who will you give me to?" At first his father would not reply, but Nachiketa persisted with the question. Since the old man had recently been pondering on the mysteries of death, he muttered angrily, "I give you to the god of death."

Undaunted, Nachiketa marched off and after much effort and hardship, found the palace of Yama, the God of death. Who would seek out and willingly go to Death before their time?

Yama, who is also called Dharmaraja or lord of the law, was away and so Nachiketa waited, fasting and praying. Three days later when Death in his awful form returned to find a fearless boy standing at his palace gates, he was pleased with the lad's devotion and determination – after all, who would seek out Death and wait for this return?... this was a rare courage.

"Since you have waited for three days I shall grant you three boons," he told Nachiketa.

"First, let my father be happy when I return to him on earth," requested Nachiketa. "Granted," answered Yama. "Next tell me how to get to heaven?" asked Nachiketa. Yama then taught Nachiketa how to attain the sorrow-less world called heaven.

Finally, the boy asked Death to explain what happens to a man after he dies, because he wanted to attain to the deathless state. Yama, was taken aback, and reluctant to reveal such secrets to a mortal. "Ask for anything else, herds of cattle, many elephants, gold, palaces and a long life." He urged.

"Oh no, I don't want any of these things!" Nachiketa persisted. "Tell me - does a man continue to exist after he dies?"

Finally, after his best efforts to change the boy's mind had failed, Yama was convinced of Nachiketa's keen desire to understand the mysteries of life and death, and assented to instruct him further.

"The soul continues to exist though the body dies and decays," explained Yama, "it is like a rider and your body is like a chariot. Your intelligence is the charioteer and your thoughts and feelings are the reins. Your five senses - sight, hearing, smell, taste and touch are the five horses that draw the chariot. The world around you is like the pastures on which these horses graze."

Then Yama taught Nachiketa the importance of Yoga. He explained how by practicing Yoga, the aspirant can bring his senses under control just as a charioteer brings his horses under control. As soon as one has controlled the senses, one will see the soul and experience the true Self. Nachiketa was the best disciple Death ever had and learnt well what Yama taught him. He made a deep effort to achieve his true nature and achieved Self-Realization, becoming a perfected being.

I would like to present Nachiketa as an ideal of a Hero to all of you for he conquered not only death, but the fear of death as well. Further, he learnt the mysteries of life from Death himself.

Truth and Nothing but the Truth

As we endure through the last few weeks of the American Election process for a new president, a striking feature that has been apparent for some years has become more and more apparent – the inability or unwillingness of politicians to tell the truth. It has disillusioned many ordinary peoples and led to a pervasive atmosphere of distrust. We really should expect more of our leaders.

It is not only that they cannot tell the truth but that they are constantly outright lying. You might think that it is naïve of me to point out something so obvious and that even young people already know. However, what is more surprising is that we are expecting and allowing this to happen. Everyone starts lying from the top of the hierarchy to the bottom.

Why do they lie? To get their job and malign their opponent – look at all the negative ads from both sides of the political spectrum. To keep their jobs – deny all wrongdoing and look the other way when there is manifest cheating – look at the way the financial crisis is being handled without any culpability. These are our representatives and if they are crooks, it is because we have allowed this to happen – it is our collective responsibility to demand higher standards from our leaders and representatives.

Truth or *Sat* is one of the aspects of the Divine. As our essential nature is this same Divinity, it is against our true nature to exaggerate, pretend, distort or lie to others, or to manipulate people for our own selfish concerns. When we live in truthfulness we become anchored in the awareness of the Divine.

Why do we lie? It is because of selfishness and the fear of losing one's reputation. However, you can fool some of the people some of the time, but you can never fool your true Self anytime! Honesty with oneself is the first step towards self-

73

improvement.

Can someone achieve any self-realization or self-knowledge by lying to others and to oneself? If you tell lies, you build up a false personality, which consists of lies and you deceive yourself. If you are immersed in lying, you will never know the truth or the Divine.

I'm not expecting that our leaders are selfless or working towards their self-realization, but the basic honesty that is required and that used to be taken for granted is essential to the well-being of society. Our whole framework crumbles when our young people see that lying and cheating is the way to get ahead – this has been demonstrated by our political, business and religious leaders for a few generations but has become more pronounced now.

We cannot allow this situation to continue just as we would not allow robbers to roam free in our towns and cities, we should not allow the demise of truthfulness. Just as we should make our personal effort to be truthful in our thoughts, word and deeds, we must teach others to be so. Further, we should hold accountable all those who seek to be our leaders to the same standard as we hold for ourselves. If we fail in this, then future generations will be brought up in the darkness of falsehood and there cannot be a spiritual society mired in deceit.

Every lie takes us away from our true nature which is anchored in Truth.

Focus on Asanas – Garudasana

1. Stand with feet shoulder width apart. Bend your knees slightly.
2. Bring your left leg to cross over your right, so that the thighs are together. Wrap your left foot around the back of your right leg just under the calf or around the ankle.
3. Balance yourself in this position.
4. Bend your elbows so that the forearms and hands stretch upward. Place palms together.
5. Cross your left arm over your right, resting your left arm in the inside of your right elbow.
6. Move your right forearm back toward the left and cross it in from of your left forearm, which moves slight back. Touch palm to palm, keeping your fingers extended.
7. Focus your eyes in front at the hands while squeezing together your arms and legs. Keep balanced on your right leg, arms and eyes centered, body upright and right knee facing front.
8. Return to the basic standing posture and repeat with the balancing on the opposite leg and with the right hand over the left.

Please be careful with balancing postures as they can be very strenuous and so should be done with caution – hold only for the duration you feel comfortable and remember to keep breathing. Those with high blood pressure or heart disease and those pregnant should avoid this posture.

Physically, this posture is very good for reducing stiffness in the joints, improving balance and stretching the spine from foot to head. Energetically, this posture opens up the energy channels in the pelvis, shoulders and upper back enabling the assimilation of energy released during other practice. Mentally, it helps to strengthen the resistance to stress and helps to steady the mind.

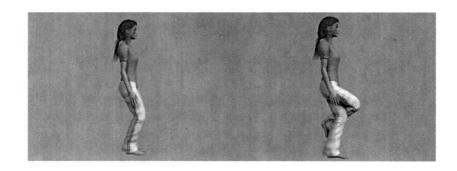

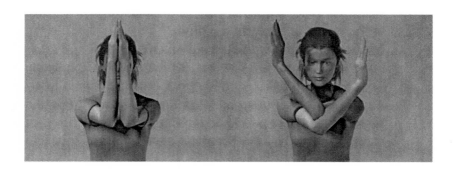

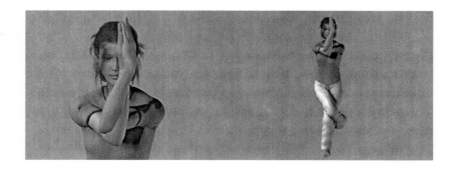

Figure 5: Garudasana

What to do with Spiritual Experiences?

Frequently, students email and ask about the experiences that they have during their practice. Should one drop the practice and flow with the visions?

Spiritual experiences can be very inspiring and help to validate that one is on the right path. However, such experiences can also be intoxicating and lead to unrealistic expectations.

It is important to keep in mind and constantly in sight the goal of our practice: Self-Realization. The objective of our practices is to remove the obstacles that prevent us from realizing our true nature and until that is accomplished, one should practice diligently and regularly as prescribed during the start or initiation into the specific path we are on. Any disruption or discontinuation of the practice is a detour from our goal and should not be entertained.

If an experience happens during practice, one should detach from it and continue with the practice. There are many such experiences of lesser or greater significance but they are all forms of distraction that can take us away from our goals. The only exception would be an ecstatic state of super-consciousness which is a state of awareness that is beyond mundane visions – an experience of this nature is beyond the mind and therefore the five senses and should not be confused with a mental experience. One need not be concerned that there would be confusion between the higher super-conscious experience and the lower mental experience – there is no way to detach from a super-conscious state and such a thought would not even be possible.

There will also be spiritual insights and experiences when one is not actively meditating – during a restful time or even during work – it can happen anytime, and is the side-effect of one's regular spiritual practice and past karmic efforts. One should learn from these experiences and give thanks for them. However, one should not form expectations or become addicted to them. One can become obsessed with insights and blissful experiences and try to duplicate them or even imagining them – this would lead to a negative mind-set if they are not recurring. What a shame it would be if someone drops away from their practice because they are not getting the vicarious experience they want!

It is also important not to fall into the trap of developing psychic powers so as to access extra-sensory experiences as these are not the fruit of one's practice and will lead to strengthening the ego, rather than realization of the true self. Psychic experiences are detours from the spiritual path and should be avoided.

In future articles, I will examine some of the major spiritual milestones which have been discussed by the Masters. Normally, it is not advisable to describe the details of the experiences because it might provide mental obstacles to their individual unfolding. There is also the danger that some spiritual seekers in their over-eagerness might simply imagine the experience in their minds – many have been fooled by their minds.
It is not my intention to be overly cautious about spiritual experiences but it is my duty to warn against being taken for a ride by the ego-mind. Enjoy yourself but don't strive or expect the experiences or try to hold on to them.

Transition For Four Years of Change

We are now rapidly approaching the end of the year 2008 and it has proved to be a transitional year, both on the material and spiritual planes. This year has heralded a great influx of spiritual energy into the mass consciousness and this has been particularly felt by those already on the path of expanding their consciousness through self-realization.

On the material plane, this year has been and continues to be one of great changes, from the election of the presidential agent of change to the world-wide collapse of the banking system. The financial system has been decimated because of a wide-spread culture of greed among our financial leaders. Hopefully, these events will lead to positive changes for the benefit of everyone. However, the short-term promises to be painful as most transitions tend to be.

We now have a president-elect who promises to make changes to the economic, health, education, political and immigration systems – in short, an overhaul of our whole way of life. Just by being elected the first black president, Barack Obama has already made a significant change to the politics of the US. His stated policy of inclusion and his straightforward and common-sense approach is a bright light in an otherwise bleak period of adversarial and negative politics.

However, the greater the promise the greater can be the disappointment and there may only be so much that one person, no matter how well-intentioned he may be, can accomplish. It is also up to all of us to help to make the changes possible. Although we are mostly focused on spiritual matters, we live in and function in the material world and so we need to consider such mundane matters as the economic conditions. Let us all send our healing energy to help our leaders make the right choices in the coming trying times. Do not underestimate the power that we can harness together.

A change in the world's consciousness will have an impact on the material plane as well, both in the positive nature, but also in creating a negative reaction in certain people. In such a way are created the agents of positive change as well as the agents of negative change. There is always a tug-of-war going on whether we are aware of it or not. Our spiritual practices and the sending of positive healing energy serve to bring positive light energy and will be very necessary for battling the forces of negativity.

There is a great deal of guidance from the Masters on the higher planes that great changes will continue for the next three years culminating in 2012, a pivotal year for the manifested world as well as the spiritual dimensions. What will happen is not revealed, but it can be for good or ill depending on all our combined efforts as well as the grace of the Masters. In the next issue, I will discuss some of the ramifications from the spiritual side which is more in our personal control.

Thanksgiving

When we awaken and open our eyes
Let us give thanks for one more day of life

When first we begin our daily practice
Let us give our thanks for the guru's grace

When we see the dawning light of the sun
Let us give thanks for spiritual guidance

As we partake of food at break of fast
Let us give thanks for divine source of all

As we perform our daily duty tasks
Let us give constant thanks to the true self

As the bright sun orb crosses mid-heaven
Let us give thanks to creative insights

As day finish and evening approach
Let us give thanks for self-less activity

When we meditate to reality
Let us give thanks to our divinity

When we ready internal fire to feed
Let us eat right and pardon the turkey
When we to bed relax body mind soul
Let us give thanks for day's lessons learned

Lord Muruga – Divine Warrior

Lord Muruga is less well-known to Westerners than Lord Ganesh, the other son of Lord Shiva. However, Lord Muruga is of great significance to spiritual practitioners of Yoga and especially kriya or kundalini yogas, as he is the lord of kundalini.

He is a direct spiritual emanation from Shiva and is called Kartikeya in North India, Subramaniam Swami in Middle India and Muruga in South India. Always depicted as a teenaged youth, he holds a spear called Vail which symbolizes the awakened kundalini and is accompanied by a peacock symbolizing the full opening of the seven chakras.

Many tales have been woven about Muruga, but the one that I wish to highlight at this time is the one where all the gods were being defeated by the host of demons and they went to Lord Shiva for help. He then placed the youth Muruga in charge of the heavenly army. Subsequently, Muruga was able to defeat the demons and restore the gods to their proper positions.

From a spiritual perspective, this story helps to illustrate the war that is fought within every one of us between the forces of light and darkness, between wisdom and ignorance. It is by harnessing the power of the awakened kundalini and the force of spiritual virtues that one can defeat the egoic and karmic negativities inherent in all of us.

All practitioners on the path are spiritual warriors – warriors of light. We must be properly armed and powered to defeat the darkness in our hearts.

The five yamas are the virtues that we must all cultivate and arm ourselves with. These are non-violence, truth, non-stealing, non-attachment and focus on the Divine. The five niyamas provide the power to overcome negativity – purity, contentment, austerity, self-study and surrender to the Divine.

The practice of kriya yoga which brings about the awakening of the kundalini energy within all of us is defined as the practice of austerity, self-study and surrender to the Divine. Therefore, the niyamas encompass the spiritual practice or sadhana that we engage in.

Since the war that we are fighting is an internal war, it does not seem as dramatic as our external wars, but nevertheless, it is more significant and difficult. If you think finding Osama Bin Laden and bringing him to justice seems to be very hard, it is nothing compared to finding the ego and putting it in its proper place!

A warrior has to train and keep fit and be able to utilize the weapons available. Everyday, the spiritual practitioner cultivates the path of light – it is a constant fight to be able to maintain a regular practice in the midst of family, work and other duties.

Let us invoke the blessings, help and guidance of the Divine Warrior – Lord Muruga, in our battles against doubt, laziness, sensuality and a host of other enemies of our spiritual evolution.

Focus On Asanas:
Warrior Pose (Virabhadrasana)

This is a great posture to prepare for the spiritual battle against negative forces. It strengthens and firms the legs, hips, and abdomen, back and neck muscles, while improving balance and concentration, as well as expanding the chest for deeper breathing. There are two parts to the asana, first a dynamic one and then a static or holding posture.

Technique:
1. Stand with feet and legs together; hands by the side.
2. Spread the feet as far apart as possible while retaining stability and keeping the heels in line with each other.
3. Inhale, raise your stretched arms overhead, keeping arms parallel. Open the chest and keep the shoulders pressed down.
4. Breathe naturally; turn your right leg and foot sideways at 90 degrees angle to the front; turn your left foot in at 45 degrees. Turn hips and body towards right. Inhale and stretch up from the waist through the arms.
5. Exhale and bend your right knee, placing the right thigh parallel to the ground. Center yourself and feel the stretch.
6. Inhale and straighten the right knee; repeat exhalation with bending and inhalation with straightening 7 times.
7. Return to position in #2 and repeat #3 through 6 with the left leg.
8. Return to position in #2 and repeat #3 through 5; now with the right knee bent, hold this position and look up towards your hands with chin reaching upward stretching the front of the neck and fingers touching. Keep your spine and back of the neck extended. Hold this for about 7 breaths and then switch to the left leg.

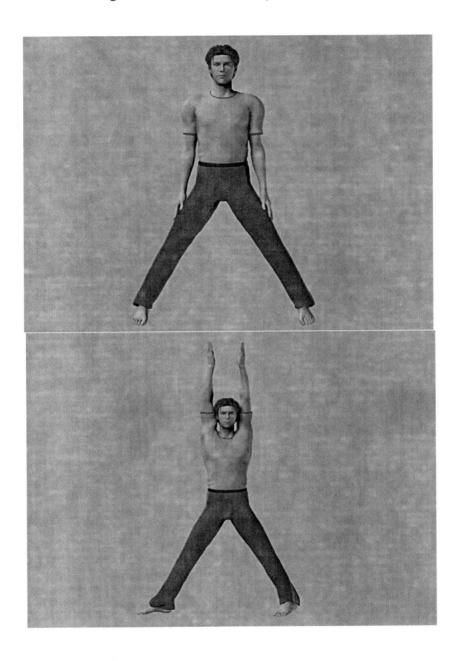

Figure 6a: Warrior Pose

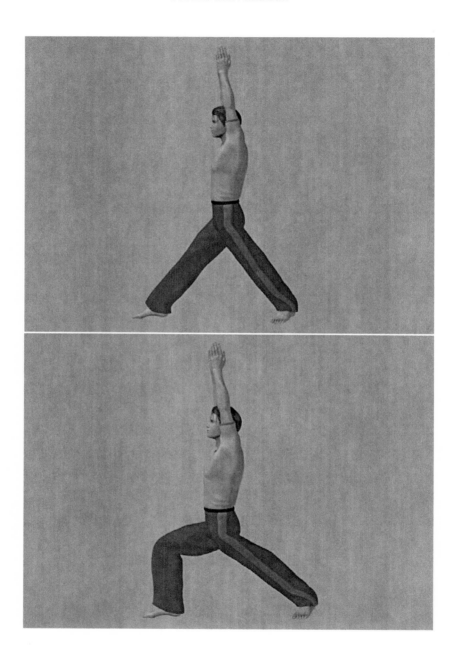

Figure 6b: Warrior Pose

Christmas

The shortest day of the year is the winter solstice on December 22nd. From the perspective of the northern hemisphere, the sun stops moving southwards around midnight of December 21st and then for the next three days appears not to move. Finally, on the 25th the sun starts to move northward again. The three days after the winter solstice are especially auspicious for meditation.

In ancient times, every year, the sun is considered to "die" on the shortest day of the year and be "reborn" three days later. This became the basis of a number of solar religions.

Spiritually, during these three days, the mystical energies are balanced and one can enter into deeper states of equanimity. I'm not advocating that you give up your celebrations and parties, only that you spend a little longer on your meditations and tune into the peaceful energies that lessen the flood of thoughts that disrupt awareness.

There is an opportunity to receive the Divine Grace for the awakening of the True Self after three days of intense meditation. In ancient times, the 3rd day after the winter solstice was celebrated by many cultures, and great "mysteries" or initiations were given on that day.

It is the day selected to be the birth day of Jesus Christ, the symbol of Super-Consciousness. It is not the day that Jesus was physically born, but the day that Jesus attained Self-Realization.

The second coming of Christ can occur to everyone of us at any time when we attain Self-Realization and eventually Divine-Realization. It is especially true on December 25th.

Some years ago, on one of my visits to Ireland, I had the opportunity to visit a stone age monument called Newgrange, which was dated to about 3300 BCE, that is 5300 years ago, much older than Stonehenge in UK. The monument was a stone mound with a long pathway leading to three chambers with stone slabs that someone could sit or sleep on. The distinctive feature of this mound is that there is above the opening a stone slit that somehow transmitted sunlight into the chambers, but only on the day of the winter solstice. However, I think that perhaps the 19th century archeologists who re-discovered it made a slight miscalculation and the chambers would have been lit 3 days later. What an experience, to meditate in the dark for 3 days and then receive the light of dawn!

Don't miss this opportunity which will occur in a few days to deepen our practice, to be re-born in the spirit.

Markandeya and Mrityunjaya

In ages past, there was an old couple who were kind and loved by one and all. However, they were secretly unhappy because they had no son. The old man, Mrikandu Munivar worshipped Shiva and sought from him the boon of begetting a son. He was given the choice between a sage with a short life on earth or a mediocre person with a long life. The couple agreed to chose the former, and was blessed with Markandeya, an exemplary son, destined to die at the age of 16.

Markandeya grew up to be a great devotee of Lord Shiva. He would travel to visit great yogis and discuss universal mysteries and truths with them. No matter where he was, every morning, after taking his bath, he would perform the worship of Lord Shiva in the form of the Shivalingam – a representation of the consciousness of the universe.

On the day of his destined death, his sixteenth birthday, Markandeya was traveling back home from another sage's hermitage. As he began his worship of Lord Shiva, the representatives of Lord Yama, the Power of Death, came to take the youth's soul, but were repulsed by the divine light surrounding him during his devotion.

The minions of Death reported the situation and Yama himself came in person to take the youth's life away. At this time, Markandeya was suddenly filled with a great dread of death, and spontaneously drew from the Divine, the great Mrityunjaya mantra and started to recite it. This mantra entreated Lord Shiva to save one from an untimely death among other blessings. When Death sprung his noose around the young sage's neck, it accidentally landed around the Shivalingam – Yama had never missed before. Shiva emerged in all his fury, and kicked Yama and killed Death itself.

The youth thanked the Lord but then entreated Him to revive Death as the death of Death would upset the world order. Lord Shiva then revived Death, but obtained his promise that the devout youth would live for ever. Another title for Lord Shiva is Mrityunjaya.

Markandeya is the seer of the Mrityunjaya mantra which saves those who recite it from untimely death. From a spiritual perspective, it can help strengthen all our positive qualities and bring more light into our lives to destroy all negative qualities.

While the day you are going to die may be pre-destined, it can be changed, but only you can change it. You yourself can bring forward the day when you are going to die through pursuing injurious habits such as drugs or smoking or even suicide, or you yourself can extend your life by earnestly expressing the demand for this extension to the Divine.

aum mrityunjaya mahādeva trāhi mām śaranāgatam
janmamityujarāvyādhi pīditam karmabandhanai

Aum, O Great Lord Mrityuñjaya,
I take refuge in You, Protect me;
And relieve me of the painful experiences of
birth, death, old-age and disease.

Seva and Sadhana

When a person finds less attraction for the fruits of the world and turns towards the spiritual world, that person becomes a spiritual aspirant. One then starts to look for a means to achieve certain spiritual goals and becomes a seeker, searching for answers to overcome unhappiness. When a seeker settles on a path he or she becomes a practitioner (sadhak) and the spiritual practice that is undertaken is called a sadhana.

My best advice is to setup a regular sadhana because it is by the once or twice daily practice that basic ignorance can be dissolved and karma overcome. It is more effective to have a short daily practice than to skip certain days and perform a long practice sporadically because karmic blockages accrue every moment. The karmic traces overlay each other and forms more linkages with the passage of time and so become more difficult to remove.

It is usually said that there is nothing more important for a sadhak than the sadhana because it is by means of the sadhana that the obstacles to eternal happiness can be removed. However, in order for the practice to progress faster, it is necessary to put aside the ego and attachment towards even the sadhana itself – it needs to be performed without expectations and desires. This of course is not truly possible until one is very much evolved.

A highly recommended way to overcome one's ego tendencies is to perform karma yoga for the sake of others or seva. This is not the charity that we do with expectations of praise or heavenly reward; it is performed selflessly without expectations or reward of any kind. It is a giving not only of material benefit, but emotional sustenance and even spiritual guidance.

Start from where you are now and decide how you can best help others. Do you have some special knowledge of some subject you can share? Do you have more wealth than is necessary for you and your family's needs and so can share some for the destitute? Use your imagination and inspiration – there is no lack of needs in this world.

For the spiritual student, one can aspire to help the spiritual teacher in spreading the awareness of the particular path and to help others on the same path. For the spiritual teacher, one can aspire to be a Servant of Humanity, not someone put on a pedestal and venerated but someone who shares and cares in the trenches with those who are suffering.

One of the great benefits of a sadhak who is a householder in the midst of the world of glitter and glass is the possibility of combining sadhana with seva – this is something that is not available to a renunciate practicing in a dark cave. Greater progress is made with seva because of the development of compassion for our brothers and sisters. Don't waste the opportunity.

Spiritual Transitioning

Previously, I had written about the focus for the year that has gone by – the expansion and development in one's spiritual practice, specifically in meditation. The focus was on controlling the mind. It is the mind which is responsible for all our suffering and it is the mind which can help us towards Self-Realization. When the mind is under the sway of the five senses, then we are on the roller-coaster of likes and dislikes and emotionally tied to the impermanent and illusive goals of material life. When one has control over the five senses, then one becomes unattached to the transient play and can then stabilize in meditation.

The focus for the coming year is on skillful action or Karma Yoga, which is activity that does not generate karmic consequences. This is possible only when there has been development in stability of the mind. In order to perfect one's activities, one needs to renounce the fruit or results from one's thoughts, words and deeds and this can only occur when one is free from all attachments. The law of causation cannot be put aside and for every action there is a reaction, but without attachment, the reaction has no hold, no means of sticking. When one takes pride or feel regret in one's actions, one takes possession for the karmic consequences – the reaction sticks.

In the beginning, one should practice by dedicating one's actions to the Divine. This does not mean that we are unconcerned about them or that the actions are performed in a mediocre manner. Without attachment, one can discharge oneself to the best of one's abilities – perform at peak level without fears or desires. You should not be concerned whether there is praise or blame, let the Divine flow through. Offer all praise to the Divine and all blame likewise – try not to react to either.

From a sadhana perspective, the focus should be on the chakras,

93

the energy centers along the spine. They are the receptacles for our karmic patterns. They affect and are effected by our thoughts, words and deeds. The six chakras correspond to different modes of activity. We are more familiar with the chakras for their roles in the awakening of kundalini shakti, but they have different levels of manifestation and should be studied and worked on for their role in the flowering of non-attachment, that is from the mental point of view.

In our personal cycle, each chakra is dominant for 30 days, during which its properties are strongest. The cycle starts in January with the muladhara or 1st chakra and moves upwards towards swadhisthana in February, manipura in March, anahata in April, vishudhi in May and the ajna or 6th chakra by June. There is also a downward cycle from July to December as the prana moves down the chakras. This annual cycle is of paramount importance for the awakening of the energy centers as well as the raising of the kundalini energy for Self-Realization.

As you discover and experience each chakra in this cycle there will be a development of greater awareness and understanding for each of them. Happy journey!

Surrender to the Divine

It is inspiring to contemplate on how one can be totally surrendered to the Divine, as this is probably something easier said than done. It would require the setting aside of our ego – that which is the subject for all aspirations, hopes, desires, attachments, sorrows, anger – that which possesses, achieves, surpasses, and plans – that which gives us our personality and defines who we are.

Can we imagine who we would be without this ego? Would we still have the same name? Would we even have a name? Can one form a relationship without the ego? Is there any point in living without hopes or desires?

There is the fear that when we are totally surrendered to the Divine, than we would lose our individuality and be a non-entity. However, this fear has no basis because it is against all precedence – we can examine the lives of those who have achieved liberation and Self-Realization. We find that they all had exemplary ideals and had miraculous achievements without the need for an ego-self.

Look at the achievements of Shakyamuni Buddha, or Jesus Christ, Adi-Shankaracharya, , Lahiri Mahasaya, Ramakrishna Paramhansa or Ramana Maharishi. Although their teachings are consistent with each other, they all had their own distinctive interpretations. It is because the Divine is infinite and multidimensional and when realized in our 3-dimensional world, the manifestation will reflect some particular facets determined by the yogi's pre-liberation interests and the time, circumstances and culture in which they had to teach.

Also, we know that these realized yogis in there exalted consciousness still knew who they had been and knew their relatives and friends and so the extinguishing of the ego did not result in an amnesiac condition. Another distinctive mark was the great Love for humanity they all shared – they did not become cold and uncaring, but in fact would even give their all including in some cases their lives for others.

We cannot understand the state of consciousness of someone like the Buddha or Jesus Christ, but we can learn something from their words and teachings which have been reported to us. Consider Jesus' words in the Lord's prayer: *"Thy will be done on earth as it is in heaven."* In the higher realms, the beings are more in tune with the Divine will and their actions reflect the correct and righteous course to be taken mostly. In our earthly realm, our egoic tendencies block our intuition of the Divine will and so most of the time, they are based on our own karmic fears and desires, that is our karmic programs. Jesus was trying to teach his disciples to learn how to put aside their individual wills and let the Divine will work through them – that is surrendering themselves to the Divine.

Obviously, there must be some practical methods that can lead to the exalted state where the Divine breathes, thinks, speaks and acts through us – yes, that is what it really means when we are talking about a being who has surrendered to the Divine. It is totally out of our normal experience or expectations and would seem a ridiculous goal at this stage. However, there is a beginning for everything (except for the Divine Nothing), and the best place to begin is where you are at present!

There are practical steps that can be taken right now to set on the path towards the state of surrendering to the Divine. A journey begins from its first step – review your relationship with the Divine. Is there a relationship and how would you describe it? It is important to formulate your relationship whether it is from your view of it now or something you would like to aspire to. Is this a servant-Master relationship, a Father-son/daughter, a

Mother-son/daughter, a Friend-friend or Teacher-student? Start from that and look at how you can strengthen the relationship or change it.

Contemplate on the obstacles that are preventing you from forming a strong and loving relationship with the Divine. Many lay blame on the Divine for the problems of this world without understanding that it is humanity who is collectively responsible for the wars and suffering on earth. We've been given a great opportunity to live on this planet but have misused our powers to bring misery to ourselves and others - don't blame the Divine and instead seek to personally change a little bit of the world for the better. Ask the Divine to help you in achieving individual peace so as to bring about social harmony.

Focus On Asanas:
Advanced Warrior Pose

The previous version of Virabhadrasana helps to build up the strength necessary to do the advanced posture with balancing on one leg.

1. Stand with your left leg in front and bent to form a right angle; thigh is parallel to the ground and arms at the side.
2. Inhale and raise your arms and fingers forward and up, with arms next to your ears as you reach through your fingers. Head and eyes face forward; shoulders pressed down.
3. Exhale and bend forward from the hips as you reach forward with your arms, bringing torso and arms parallel to the ground. Keep right leg extended with your foot planted on the ground. Inhale and feel the stretch between arms and right leg.
4. Exhale and shift weight forwards over your left foot and leg. Eyes looking down to the ground. Raise your right leg, keeping it extended with toes pointing out behind you, parallel to the ground. Feel the stretch between the fingers and the right foot. Maintain the pose and breathe normally.
5. Exhale, return to starting position. Switch legs so that you now have the right leg in front and bent to form a right angle. Repeat steps 2 to 4.

Besides strengthening the legs and spine, this posture also improves balance and concentration, as well as strengthening the ears and eyes.

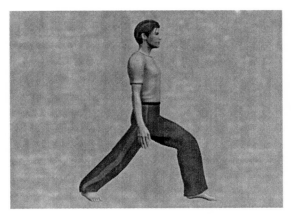

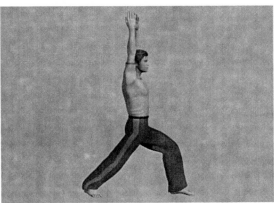

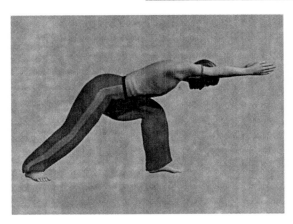

Figure 7a: Advanced Warrior Pose

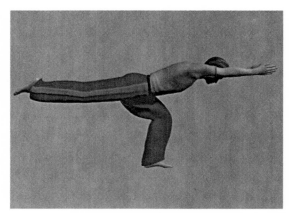

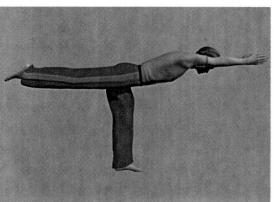

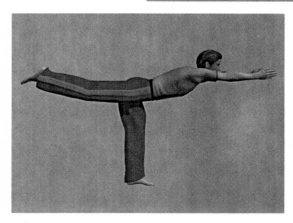

Figure 7b: Advanced Warrior Pose

Desire Is The Source
Of Our Suffering

The 2nd energy center or swadhisthana chakra is the center for attraction and aversions. We are attracted to certain things and people and have an aversion for others. The specifics are governed by our present and past karmic patterns – our urges and compulsions.

The 2nd center is responsible for the instinct to preserve our species, that is for reproduction. However, nowadays, this urge is no longer needed as much as before, but it is just as strong if not more than ever.

Unlike animals, which just express their urges in a straightforward manner, "the pinnacle of evolution on earth" has misused his imagination to create an unending number of objects, situations and experiences to try to indirectly satisfy these urges. We have created all sorts of conditions and criteria for food – the look, taste, texture and smell. There arises the myriad desire for status, power and accumulation of possessions and lust for satisfaction of the senses.

Emotional pleasure arises from the satisfaction of a desire, and an emotional dependency results from the habitual connection of pleasure with the satisfaction. Unpleasant emotions or displeasure result from the experience of situations or objects, which we would like to avoid, leading to a habitual aversion for those situations or objects. All of us have things we like and those, which we dislike, and it is not always clear how it all came about that we react within the set program.

Desires are like the ten-headed monster of legend – you cut of one-head and nine more arise and takes it place – satisfying one desire only gives rise to many more and there does not seem to be an end to them. A desire gains strength over time unless one can detach from it or transform it to another desire.

Emotions are a complex and tangled web that have many interconnected layers and various sources, but desire is one of the primary causes.

Anger arises when a particular desire is unfulfilled, and if this frustration continues, unreasoning violence in thought, word or deed, rears its ugly head. Under the constraints of modern society, anger is suppressed, leading to stress, a leading cause of ill health such as high-blood pressure or mental illnesses. There are those schools of thought that promote the release of "negative emotions", supposing that such cathartic exercises would release stress and promote a positive effect. Aside from leaving a person drained for a certain period, and therefore incapable of further emotional outbursts for that period, no long-term benefit seems to occur. The positive experience seems to indicate that it is the channeling of the emotional power, which is valuable, that has long-term effects, and should be pursued.

Jealousy and envy arises when our desires are fulfilled by others. We begin to long for or covet the experiences or possessions of those who seem to "have it all". Such a reaction arises when we feel an emptiness within ourselves, caused by our inability to connect with our Center, the Divine within us, the True Self. There is no desperate grasping for external validation when one feels the inner completion, the joy of Self-realization.

To get rid of all desires is practically unfeasible and only theoretical talk of those who do not practice. Instead, one of the best ways to deal with desires is to channel all of them into one great desire. Of course, it would be best if that primary desire is a very positive one, such as the desire for Self-Realization. Just as one does not need a bridge once we get across the river, so also, even this grand desire will disappear once satisfied!

There are many stories that help to illustrate how desires can be helpful to liberation. Consider the case of the young man who was in love with a beauty who did not reciprocate and spent his days being love-lorn and in despair. He appealed to Lord Krishna to help him win his love. However, when Lord Krishna appeared to him, the Lord made light of the youth's beloved lady. The young man kept praising the lady's beauty until Lord Krishna showed him the beautiful nymphs of heaven who made the earth lady seem unattractive in comparision. A great desire now arose in the youth for the heavenly ladies and he begged Lord Krishna to satisfy this desire. The Lord then instructed him in the appropriate spiritual practice that would enable him to reach the heavenly realms. The enthusiastic youth spurred on by his inflamed desire practised day and night and soon reached high states of consciousness. One night he found himself transported to the abode of Lord Krishna - he had overshot the heavenly realms where the nymphs were and reached the higher heavens where such sensual pleasures were not indulged in. The youth was quite disappointed!

Don't Let Fear Rule You

Everyone thinks they know all about fear but few ever think about it, trying to avoid it as much as possible. The fact is that this emotion is so basic that it is almost impossible to become free from it. Fear arises from the instinct of self-preservation which was very important in the early days of humanity. We needed to react to mortal threats with the flight or fight program in those primitive times. However, we are still under the same programming without the same stimuli – there are no saber-tooth tigers hunting us these days. The fear of death is one of the most enduring one that a human possesses.

It is the lesser variations of fear which dominate in modern times – stress and tension. Fear comes and goes – if you see someone point a gun at you, fear may grip your heart but when he puts the gun away, fear is relieved. However, stress is like background music, it is always there. We have little means to release stress because we are not even aware that it is there because we have become used to it. Paradoxically, only when one has attained complete relaxation does one recognize the encroachment of stress.

We do not require an immediate threat to feel some mode of fear because we have evolved beyond animal consciousness to human consciousness. The blessings of imagination and thinking ahead, which animals do not possess to any degree have the double-edged consequence of causing stress. When a person thinks about the consequence of his action or inaction, such as being late for work or an important meeting, stress is increased. If you imagine yourself losing your job, more stress will spoil your life, but is it an immanent danger that requires such a reaction? We are doing it from habit and cannot stop.

We have been programmed from infancy to react with fear to certain stimuli. It is the punishment and reward system in the family, school, work and society that habituates us to fear the results of failure (however that is defined.) Even when success is achieved in a certain activity, the process has set up so much stress already that we cannot even enjoy the relief.

Tragically, there is even a fear of the unknown. It creates another level of stress that adds to the fear of death. Imagine a stress cake with many layers – the bottom layer is the fear of death and then additional layers are piled on based on our situation.

There is such an emotional perversion that we seek out "harmless" situations that can excite our imagination with horror and fear. Have we ever wondered why so many people actually go and watch horror movies so that they can get scared? The reason that fear and stress can become so habitual is because there is an adrenaline rush when we get scared – remember the flight or fight instinct that we have from our evolutionary past.

I would recommend that you contemplate the various kinds of fears and how they arise. Meditate on how stress is affecting your life and what it would feel like if you were totally relaxed and unaffected by fears.
Examine your life-style and mark down those activities that are contributing to your stress level. It might be a good idea to change or even omit these activities in the future. Don't think that we can't change things – make the effort now.

Ethics and Self-Realization

In ancient times the sages emphasized the development and practice of ethics above all as the pre-eminent spiritual practice. However, in present times this has become unfashionable and there is much greater emphasize on the Guru's grace or in the effectiveness of techniques. It is understandable because the effect of grace or the techniques are more apparent while that of morality is difficult to ascertain from our worldly perspective.

Is there any harm in neglecting the development of moral character as part of one's spiritual practice?

Effective spiritual practices which lead to self-realization have to release the past karmas so that they can be either worked out positively or removed by further practice. However, such a release usually gives rise to emotional or mental reactions that can cause new karmic consequences. For example, memories of past traumas can give rise to emotions such as anger or despair and if one cannot detach from such emotions, they will be expressed outwardly against another person, thereby causing new negative karma. In this example, the spiritual practice, rather than help in progressing towards less karma would increase one's karmic burden instead – a step backward.

When you are firmly grounded in positive virtues such as truthfulness and harmlessness, then you can easily process all the "stuff" that come out from your practice without being negatively effected. Rather than an emotional catharsis which causes more emotional ripples around, you would be able to release the negativity by detachment or transformation.

Transforming a negative emotion such as anger into a positive emotion such as love takes practice and does not happen automatically. That is the reason why we must form ethical habits and the moral injunctions such as those given by Patanjali in his Yoga Sutras are a reminder that they are necessary.

Living life under these ethical rules helps to generate the behavior patterns that will enable us to deal with the unfolding of our karmic burdens successfully. From a subtle perspective, our nadis and chakras are purified through them so that the chakras can be awakened. Only after the chakras are awakened and the nadis purified is it prudent to awaken the kundalini energy.

Please do consider the importance of ethical rules in your spiritual life – it will smooth out a lot of the negative events in the practitioner's life.

The Chakras - Keys To Health And Spiritual Evolution

Why do I put so much emphasis on the chakras in my teachings?

There is probably no other yogic tool as important as that of the energy centers or chakras since they have important roles for both the physical, emotional and mental health of a person as well as being pivotal in attaining to higher conscious states.

There are hundreds of chakras in the energy body but the six major ones along the subtle spine are the most crucial. This is because they are the repositories of our karma. The six chakras are the muladhara at the perineum (connected to the base of the spine), swadhisthana at the sacrum (about 3 inches above the base), manipura at the back corresponding to the navel, anahata or heart center, vishuddhi at the base of the neck and ajna in the middle of the brain. There is of course the 7th chakra called sahasrara chakra or thousand-petalled lotus at the top of the head but this center is that of perfection and does not have any function.

It is very useful to learn the names of the chakras themselves as they have mantric significance and the repetition of their names causes vibrations at the energy centers.

Each of the chakras is responsible for certain bodily functions – the muladhara is responsible for the physical body as a whole, the swadhisthana for the emotional body, the manipura for the energy body, the anahata for the mental body and the vishuddhi for the causal body.

There is also overlapping of functionalities in that although muladhara has overall control of the physical body, it also has minor functions for emotions, energy, mental states and karmic memory. For instance, this first chakra rules the emotions of fear and courage.

It is important to understand that these energy centers are very subtle pranic structures and are maintained directly by the life-force energy. When the life-force energy is depleted, then they cannot function properly and then every aspect of our life that they control will be hurt. On the flip side, when we do, say or even think something negative which resonates with a particular chakra, then it becomes depleted of prana! Of course when we apply ourselves positively, then more prana will go to the chakra concerned.

In the subtle energy body, the chakras are connected together by fine filaments of energy called the nadis. These nadis act like the arteries and nerves in the physical body, and they can be blocked or even damaged so that some parts of the subtle body might not be getting the life-force needed. However, since they are energy filaments, they can be repaired, redirected and even grown by the power of prana – this aspect is essential for healing purposes.

For the spiritual evolution and development of higher consciousness, the main energy channel called sushumna nadi flows along the spine and through the 6 major chakras that we have been discussing. It is through this central channel that the latent kundalini shakti has to rise up for the bliss of samadhi and the flowering of super-conscious states. Therefore, each chakra has to be sufficiently opened and filled with life-force energy before the kundalini will be attracted up to it. We need to work progressively upward in the normal course of events in order to raise the kundalini but in practical safety terms, it is recommended to try to open the 6th chakra or ajna first, in order to provide the positive pull from above.

If the higher chakras are shut and we open up the lower ones, then there may be difficulties encountered in the first three chakras which may challenge the practitioner's ability to cope. There are practices which work on all 6 chakras progressively without over-emphasizing on any one at a time and these are the kind of practice that I recommend. Even when one is putting greater emphasis on one particular chakra in order to work out certain problems, it is always a good idea to exercise all the other chakras regularly to some extent. For instance, if you are spending half an hour on the heart chakra, combine it with a five minute each practice on the other five chakras, making up almost an hour.

Working on the chakras is a life-long pursuit but one of the most worthwhile that anyone can embark on. The healing affects can occur very quickly but due to our karmic inertia and habit patterns, the energy centers cannot be so easily opened and developed for spiritual purposes. However, it is a necessity for Self-Realization and so persevere in your efforts.

The Future Is In Our Own Hands

As I watched the inauguration of President Obama a couple of days ago, it occurred to me how much hope and expectation is being invested onto a single individual. Collectively, the whole nation seemed to be wishing that all our troubles will dissipate with the departure of the outgoing president and that a new age is dawning with the change in leadership.

Of course there are many important decisions that only a president can make and they will affect our lives for years to come. Let us leave him to do his work and pray for the best from our leaders.

I'm not advocating that we simply sit back and watch the unfolding drama, thinking that our duty ended with his election. It is time to remember that we are each ultimately responsible, personally and collectively, for what happens in this world and cannot blame nor adulate our political or spiritual leaders beyond a certain point.

We also have a responsibility for what happens around us - how we help or refuse to aid those in need when confronted with the opportunity. How we discharge our obligations to family, friend, society and the world. We are familiar with our duties to our family and friends, although some have sought to hide from them – for example, fathers who don't take responsibilities for their children – which create negative ripples that go beyond the current generation.

Our responsibility for society and the world is less clear – it seems so remote and large and we do not seem to have any direct relationship to them. If there is a relationship, it seems to work the other way, changes in society or the world impact us. What can we do that can effect the larger aspect of our existence? In order to understand this, we must first distinguish between that which happens to us and our reaction to that which happens.

We do not have much control on external circumstances but have total control over how we deal with them. When we refuse to accept falsehood and the harming of innocent people, we setup the vibration around us that can help to strengthen the resolve of those who are wavering in their ethical stand and willing to compromise their morality. This is just one example.

Remember that the choices you make now will determine who you will be in the future. You can choose to let life dictate who you are or you can choose to overcome your predispositions. Instead of taking the easy road, take the right path to achieve your goals. Let your leaders know in no uncertain terms what is acceptable and what is not. Be a good example for your family and friends by developing a loving attitude – let go of anger in your reactions. Develop a spiritual practice and burn-up your karma which is limiting you from achieving freedom from your emotional behavior patterns.

Focus On Meditation:
The Senses Of Smell & Taste

The senses of smell and taste are associated with the 1st and 2nd chakras respectively. The control of these senses is necessary for the awakening of these two chakras. Normally, we are under their spell and do not really understand what they are doing unless challenged by strong stimuli such as a perfume or some chilly food.

In the first meditation, connect the appropriate chakra with a sense, for example, the 1st chakra and smell. Take some real smell such as a rose or an essential oil and let the aroma fill you while concentrating on the chakra. Do this for at least 10 minutes.

Next, imagine a specific aroma and try to "smell" it – this will be difficult for many people, but can be developed just as visualization can be developed for the sense of sight.

Practice for at least 10 minutes. Take a particular smell and stick to it for some period of time instead of changing it every meditation session.

In the third meditation, try to vary the aroma in a session – you can try to imagine three to five related smells. Practice for 10 minutes.

For the first 4 weeks, practice to control the sense of smell and then change to the sense of taste for another 4 weeks.

Can There Be
Satisfaction In This Life?

Greed is one of the emotions associated with our navel chakra. At the first chakra, the almost omnipresent desire for life gives rise to the instinct for survival while in the second chakra it gives rise to the instinct to reproduce. In the third chakra, there is the desire to control our environment including other people. This gives rise to all the efforts to shelter from the elements and to ensure a dependable food supply.

Over time, the simple desire to control our environment has given over to more complex urges to accumulate possessions beyond necessity, giving rise to greed. After all, how much money does one need to live a comfortable life? How big a house, how expensive a car, how much jewelry and how many wives or husbands? It appears there is no answer and like the gobbling monsters of nightmares and video-games, the mouth is huge and always ready to swallow some more.

The sad fact is that greed prevents us from finding satisfaction in our lives. There cannot be contentment because we have been brought up as a consumer society and greed is actually encouraged – the loud voice says that the one who dies with the most wins, even though, a tiny whispering voice warns that you cannot take it with you.

We are discontented when we see someone else with more than us and we would like to take it away from them. Everything has a range of bigger, better, prettier, more expensive, rarer etc. etc. to lure one into desiring after it. How many cars can you drive at one time? Does one person really need a dozen cars?

Amazingly, greed is not limited to material things. Spiritual students can become greedy for more and more spiritual techniques and can accumulate many more than they can possibly practice and still pine for more. Some become greedy for spiritual experiences and journey here and there to get something from this Master or that one.

The antidote to greed is contentment and a feeling of abundance. We need to detach from envy and desire for possessions beyond necessity. Find a middle path – you don't have to limit yourself to a grass hut if it is in your means to live in a sturdy house in a good neighborhood. The danger of greed is going beyond your need or beyond your means. If you obtain something that you cannot afford, it will cause misery down the road. Be contented and happy with what you have – this is an active meditation that has to be done constantly. Visualize yourself as you are now, with what you have now and see yourself being happy and contented. Don't wait for the pot of gold at the end of the rainbow before you try to be contented – these illusory goals are mirages that disappear when you approach them. Do it now.

The Dawning of the Age of Aquarius

Like the song says, it is the dawning of the age of Aquarius, or is it? When do we really enter this much awaited age and what does it mean for us?

Unfortunately, the only thing all experts are agreed on is that they all disagree on the timing of this new age. Some say that we are already there while others put the event several hundred years in the future. There are several factors involved that is causing this confusion. First, the exact length of a zodiac age is unsure and the other is the exact point at which a constellation is said to start a new age. These uncertainties are due to the different ways of measuring the ending and beginning edges of a sign in the zodiac.

The zodiacal age is based on the constellation which is in the skies on the spring equinox or March 21st. The zodiac wheel consists of twelve constellations making up around twenty five thousand one hundred years, with each constellation averaging around two thousand one hundred and fifty years. However, the constellations have different sizes and so the ages vary in length. The exact sizes of the constellations have only been determined less than one hundred years ago. In the past, it was estimated by eye and so an age may have started for one or two hundred years or even more before it was seen visually. Thankfully, there is considered to be an overlap of two hundred years when one age ends and another begins.

These twelve constellations have been given different characteristics by the ancient observers and we are still following their model. So each age takes on the characteristics of the constellation that it is named after. We have been or are still in the age of Pisces or the Fish constellation. This may have started over two thousand years ago and we should be at the tail-end of it. During this period, major religions have arisen because of the pull of Pisces while materialism and focus on sexuality has arisen because of the pull from its opposing sign Virgo.

What will the age of Aquarius bring? It should bring technology, worldwide organizations and more focus on humanity while the opposing sign Leo will bring about global warming and a focus on even greater individuality and global dictators. Not exactly the age of peace that the song sings about necessarily. Of course it is over two thousand years long and there could be lots of things going on.

The change into a new age also involves the coming of an avatar or messiah. The new age will bring the Kalki Avatar or Maitreya Buddha or the 2nd Coming of Christ. When this happens or whether these will be a single Being or multiple ones is not clear. This great Being does not come at the beginning of the age necessarily and will be preceded by his helpers who are either ascended Masters or even avatars or Divine incarnations in their own right.

However, it seems to me that rather than waiting for such earth-shattering events to occur, we have the means to bring about our own ideal age through our own efforts. This is what yogic spiritual practice is all about. If we can bring about our own higher consciousness, and then lead others to do so as well, then the world's consciousness is lifted up to a certain degree which can then lead to changes in society, politics, education and so on.

The Last Days Now?

A few days ago, I watched a movie about the "end of days," a popular theme that has been frequently done in the last thirty years, most famously with the "Omen" series. In this genre of Christian movies, the agency is some sort of "Anti-Christ" who needs to come to fulfill some sort of gruesome prophecy involving the death of millions. In the more secular versions, we have the disaster movies which involve meteors, asteroids, comets, earthquakes or aliens.

What's the attraction to imagining an end of the world scenario? There is a deep down acknowledgement that the world is messed up and no amount of human effort is going to fix things and so why not put an end to it and start over again? This may have something to do with our basic dissatisfaction with ourselves and what we have done – it is the deep desire to push the "reset button" on life, to start over again. There may also be a primal fear from the subconscious layer of the mind which has traces of ancient mega-disasters on earth. Whatever the reasons, besides making money for Hollywood, we can also take advantage of these thoughts.

Let us imagine that the world is going to end in one day, or a week and we are going to die.

What would you do different from what you are doing now? Would you still go to work tomorrow? Would you contact your family and friends and say goodbye? Would you do more meditation or would you rent more videos and have a movie marathon? Would you stay in bed and feel sorry for yourself or contact your former best friend whom you haven't talked to in ten years because of a trivial argument? Or would you keep doing what you are doing now?

Try writing out a 24 hour plan and a week-long plan.

The world may not end in the foreseeable future but it could end for us personally anytime. No one knows when that day will come. When we wake up in the morning, we should thank the Divine for another day of life and make the most of it. Normally, people live like their life will last forever and never give a thought to death. However, for some people there is a rude awakening when some life-threatening situation such as a serious disease occurs or some serious accident – a brush with death often motivates people into a spiritual perspective. Why wait for something to happen?

Make a daily plan for yourself that you would stick to even if you only had one day to live! Maximize the opportunity of this uncertain life-span and never have to regret.

The Personal Significance of MahaShivaratri

On February 23rd, we celebrated what is popularly called the Day of Shiva. There are many stories about what the significance of this day is to spiritual seekers. Whatever story they subscribe to, there is no disagreement among yogis and Shiva devotees that it is the holiest day of the year for them. Many will fast for twelve or twenty-four hours over the night with chanting and ritual worship of the shivalinga. A very few will meditate and perform their spiritual practice as an offering to the Lord.

From the cosmic perspective, it is the day marking symbolically when Lord Shiva acquired his blue throat. At the time of creation, the gods and demons were co-operating to churn the cosmic ocean of milk in order to produce the nectar of immortality. However, during this process, a pot of poison which could have unmade all of creation came out and the terrified gods went to Lord Vishnu, the preserver of creation for a solution. The Lord Vishnu advised them to seek the aid of Lord Shiva, who alone could save them. Out of compassion for creation, Lord Shiva drank the poison and by his power, held it in his throat (turning it blue) without letting it go into his stomach. The gods and demons chanted and danced His glory all day and night in celebration.

From a microcosmic perspective, there is the story of a hunter who got lost in the jungle and climbed a bael tree as evening approached so as to escape from the wild animals roaming in the night. In order to keep from falling asleep and falling off the tree, he plucked a leaf every now and then, intoning "Om Nama Shivaya." At the same time, his water bottle was leaking water down the tree. In the morning he gave thanks to the Lord and went home to his family. Before he could eat his meal, a stranger came knocking on the door and as required by rules governing proper behavior, he gave food to the guest before eating himself.

Throughout his life, he was blessed with ample supply of food and a happy family. At the time of his death, two messengers of the Lord came and took him to the abode of Lord Shiva where he dwelled in bliss for eons, before taking birth again on earth as a great king. All this came about because without his knowledge, there was a buried shivalinga under the tree where he had sought refuge and so he was actually giving worship to the Lord throughout the night as he dropped bael leaves and water on it. Also, he fed someone else before he broke his fast in the morning.

When Lady Parvati asked Lord Shiva which day was most auspicious to worship him to receive his blessings, the Lord responded that the 14th day of the new moon of the last lunar month of the year was dearest to him. This occurs around February or March of the solar calendar.

Do these stories have any significance for us personally?

The first story teaches us that with our spiritual practice, there will be produced lots of toxic emotional and mental poison that will need to be transformed before the nectar of immortality or Self-Realization can be achieved. Only by the grace of the Lord and the appropriate practices can the process be completed. The day or night of Mahashivaratri is particularly auspicious for the transforming of our negativities into the bliss of super-consciousness. One must remember this during the celebration and practice sessions.

The second story helps us to understand that any amount of practice even if we are distracted will be helpful for our spiritual growth. After all, even when the worship was done accidentally, the fruit and grace was granted! It is useful to remember that those who have not had the opportunity to receive a spiritual practice rely on external worship for betterment of their lives and to obtain better re-births. Those who are spiritual practitioners rely primarily on their practice instead of external worship, although they can also benefit from appropriate rituals. This knowing that we can not really mess up with our practices as long as we do them with sincerity and to the best of our abilities is indeed comforting and is worth celebrating on at least one special day a year.

What Do The Eyes See ?

We are totally dependent on our five senses and would be lost without them. Of all the senses, the one that we rely on most is our vision. But how much of reality do we really see with our eyes?

It is instructive to consider the limitations of our vision in relation to our understanding of the world and reality in order to better appreciate the teachings of the yogis. Our eyes have a limited range of light frequencies that it can sense, that is the visible light range and we have to depend on scientific instruments to detect and map out higher frequencies such as ultra-violet and x-rays as well as lower frequencies such as infra-red and radio waves. Although we cannot see them, they can have detrimental effects on our bodies and we would not necessarily even feel their effects immediately, but only after some damage has been done. The eyes can warn us of some dangers such as wild animals and gun toting thieves, but is helpless against these "invisible" dangers.

Our eyes cannot see very small objects and so we need microscopes to detect bacteria and atoms. Look at a nearby wall or the ground that you are standing on – looks pretty solid doesn't it? However, physics tell us that all matter is made up of atoms which have tiny electrons whizzing around a small solid nucleus and in fact is almost all empty space. Our eyes and sense of touch cannot detect this empty space. An atom is so empty that as an illustration, we can imagine an empty football stadium with a ball in the center and some tiny marbles whizzing around it throughout the field. We cannot see this with our limited vision and think that matter is solid. The yogis by the superior vision that does not rely on their eyes have penetrated to reality and so consistently teach us that the world is an illusion.

The yogis are telling us that the world that we think we see is not really what is actually there because what we see is limited by our vision and is just a projection – that is an illusion.

We see three dimensions and suppose the world is three dimensional, but in fact when external light penetrates our eyes, a two dimensional image is formed in our retina and it is by mental process that a three dimensional image is formed from multiple two dimensional images from two eyes. We cannot form a four or five dimensional image and even the three dimensions is another projection. What does the world really look like?

You might think that we could use instruments to help us penetrate reality but that is still in its early stages, limited by the technology as well as our minds to design the right instruments since we cannot imagine anything higher than three dimensions. Although our mathematics has been able to do so for several hundred years, there are too many unknowns and variables for us yet to be able to visualize it and in fact we may not be able to without accessing our higher vision which is independent of our eyes and the rest of the optical apparatus.

If we can actually see what we look like to each other we might be surprised and gladdened into uttering "Namaste," that, "I bow to the indwelling Spirit within you." The yogis have taught that we are not just the physical body but have bodies of finer and subtler matter and that we are actually spirit informing matter. However, we cannot see the subtle matter and we have not yet developed instruments which can detect this subtle matter. The only instrument capable of discerning reality at this time is the superior awareness vision of super-consciousness, which can only be developed by the practice of spiritual techniques given by the ancients.

Focus On Mudra:
To Counter Exhaustion and Dizziness

The following mudra is very effective for recharging one's energy reserves and to center oneself. It is called Rudra Mudra and draws strength and energy from the navel center and counteracts general weakness.

It should be practiced with both hands holding the gesture without tension for about 5 minutes and can be repeated three times. One should sit comfortably if possible rather than lying down, but in a situation where there is dizziness, one can lean against a bed or wall.

Place the tips of your thumb, index finger and ring finger together, while extending the other fingers without tension.

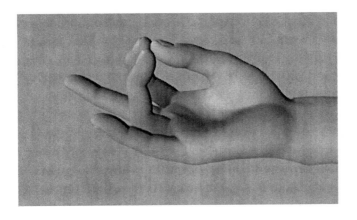

Figure 8: Rudra Mudra for Energization

Chakra and Consciousness

In the evolution of consciousness there is a corresponding activation and opening of the pranic energy centers called chakras.

From the first base chakra (muladhara) to the navel chakra (manipura) spans the domain of animal consciousness. The so-called unconscious mind of instincts reside in the first chakra while the subconscious mind of impressions and past-life programming or samskaras reside more in the 2nd and 3rd chakras. From this one can realize how deep and strongly embedded are the instincts for survival and reproduction within our chakra system. From the instinct of survival arise the fight or flight response which is accompanied by the fear complex of feelings and emotions, while from the reproduction instinct has arisen the feelings of lust and emotions of desire.

In the 3rd chakra, we see the first glimmerings of individuality, but still from a subconscious level with the focus on the instinct of hunger becoming a thirst for accumulation of possessions - from the instinct of survival we seek to control our environment with a roof over our head and a supply of food stored away. From the instinct of reproduction we now seek to control our mate (s) and satisfy our pleasure sensations whenever we wish. The manipura chakra is the abode of greed.

Of course, you may wonder that I've talked about the negatives of these three chakras without giving any of their positives, for surely they have their counterpoints to balance them. In actuality, the first two chakras have no negatives – they are natural and animalistic – the negative feelings and emotions come from the impact of our evolved individuality on these first two chakras. In a way, it is our developing human consciousness that has perverted the unconscious and sub-conscious.

The 4th chakra is the heart chakra or anahata wherein our conscious mind resides – this is the meeting point between the lower animal consciousness and the higher divine consciousness. Here are all the good and bad, for here is where we differentiate ourselves from others and take animal instincts into excess and even perversions – here is where we turn simple hunger into excessive indulgence and obesity and simple sex into rape and pornography. Paradoxically, this is also where our mind can turn towards our True Self, towards the Divine and achieve Divine Love and Compassion, and liberate ourselves into super-consciousness and beyond.

The fifth chakra or Vishuddhi is where super-consciousness resides. This is no longer the mind as we know it, which is limited by three dimensional space and time…limited by the domain of the five senses. Here we can experience higher dimensions of reality unconstrained by the physical body and senses. This is where we begin to communicate with our True Self. It is still in the realm of duality with object subject distinctions, but at its higher stages the two merge as we approach the realm of the 6th chakra or ajna.

The knowledge and practice of chakra therapy is indeed marvelous because the chakras contain our suffering in the form of karmic blocks as well as our salvation in the promise of evolution towards higher consciousness as we unravel their mysteries.

Householder Yogis

It is difficult for seekers who have family responsibilities to find the time and make the effort to achieve Self-Realization. Many dream of being able to leave their duties behind them and retire to a cave in the Himalayas. This tendency is especially fueled by stories of saints who have renounced their lives and went off to remote places to achieve liberation from the cycle of suffering.

However, it may not be widely known that these stories of external renunciation are rather recent, from about two thousand five hundred or so years ago only. This time-frame corresponds roughly to the dark age of increasing material ignorance called Kali Yuga as outlined by Shri Yukteswar in his masterpiece Divine Science. The Lord Buddha came just at the beginning of this era and gave the example of leaving his princely life behind him and seeking for his enlightenment in the wilderness. His example was a departure from the sages that had gone before him.

In an earlier age, as recorded in the ancient scriptures, we have many stories of the householder sages as exemplified by the great beings called the septa-rishis or 7 sages who are the rays of the seven stars of the Great Bear. They were all married and had family and were the head of great lineages of saints. A great example was Vashishta who was the Guru of the royal family that included the god-prince Rama. He was the greatest sage of his time and his wife considered a paragon of virtue and wisdom – she was called Arundhati and ascended to be a star just next to her husband.

Another famous example was the great sage-king Janaka who was glorified for his inner renunciation to his palaces and great wealth. His guru was sage Yagnavalkya whose wife Gargi was also renowned for her wisdom. All the great Upanishads or spiritual texts from three thousand years ago to the time of the Buddha are based on the examples of householder sages.

At the end of the this minor Kali Yuga and beginning of the more spiritual age called Dwapara, around 1862, Mahavatar Babaji initiated Lahiri Mahasaya into Kriya Yoga and started a whole new cycle for accelerated spiritual evolution. Lahiri Baba was a householder and had children after his initiation by Babaji. He never retreated from his responsibilities and discharged his duties diligently, while at the same time attaining his enlightenment and spreading the teachings of Babaji to another generation of disciples.

All spiritual seekers should keep in mind the example of Lahiri Baba when they are considering to become a vagabond yogi. It is easier to go to a cave and meditate without dealing with the vagaries and demands of the material life. It is much more difficult to balance the living of a spiritual life in the material world. However, just as a sword is tempered in fire and water, it is actually easier for the householder yogi to be truly tested and can become immune to worldly temptations. It is the development of inner renunciation that is the true renunciation exalted by the sages. Remember this the next time you wish that you had not taken on the duties and responsibilities of a family. Persevere.

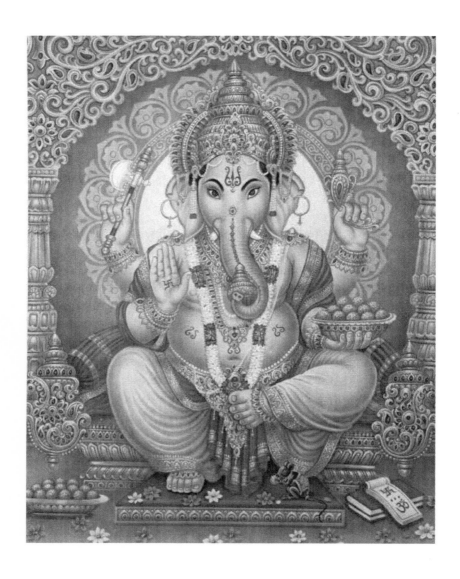

May Lord Ganesha Help Us Overcome All Obstacles On Our Path

Lord Ganesha –
Overcoming Obstacles

One of the most intriguing of all the Divine cosmic forces that can come to our aid is that of Lord Ganesha. The elephant-headed son of Lord Shiva is called Ganapati, the Lord of the ganas or heavenly host; Vinayaka, the Supreme Leader; and also as Vighneshvara, or the Lord of Obstacles. These names indicate that He is the master of the circumstances that obstruct any path and with His help, all obstacles can be overcome. This is why all auspicious acts and rituals are undertaken with His invocation first.

From a yogic point of view, Lord Ganesha as the Lord of the physical world represented by the first energy center or muladhara chakra, helps to overcome all external physical, emotional and mental obstacles.

The form of Lord Ganesha is very symbolic and it can be very instructive for us to learn more about it:

1. The large head of an elephant is necessary to hold all the knowledge that is in the universe. The elephant is also a symbol of wisdom and of long memory.
2. The big ears are for listening to scriptures and to hear our pleas for help.
3. The trunk is a very versatile instrument – it can be used to lift heavy objects or a fine blade of grass. Our intellect should be able to be so efficient that we can solve all the problems, big or small that occur in our lives.
4. There are two tusks to indicate that we should be able to differentiate between good or evil, right or wrong, real or unreal. However, one tusk is broken to indicate that we should grow out of the world of relativity based on pairs

of opposites to achieve unity.

5. His vehicle is a mouse which represents desire – it is very small but capable of much damage if not under control. The mouse looks at the food placed before Lord Ganesha, but does not eat without His permission.

6. In one hand He holds a rope which is used to pull us towards Him, while in a second hand, He holds an axe to cut off our harmful desires. In a third hand, he holds a sweet rice ball to reward those that reach towards Him and in the fourth hand, He blesses them.

7. In a side view, He has the outline of the Sanskrit character of OM – the essential vibration of the universe.

The following is a mantra for invoking his presence and blessings:

Suklaambaradaram Vishnum
Shashi-varnam Caturghujham
Prasanna vadanam dhyaayet
Sarva vighnopa Shantayet.

I meditate on Lord Ganesha, who wears white garments
and is all-pervading
Whose color is that of the moon, who is four-armed
Whose face is always peaceful and happy
I meditate on Him who removes all obstacles.

Love as Virtue

Emotions by definition and practical experience are evanescent and cannot be constant because they are continually affected by our thoughts. We are unable to keep an emotion for any length of time without it exhausting us and boring us.

The emotion of love is no exception in that our feelings are changing all the time with new experiences. A couple can fall in and out of love in a matter of weeks or even days. However, most mothers will love their children in spite of a myriad of reasons not to – it has been said that there are some people whom only their mothers can love!

It seems that humanity has taken something of high value and trashed it by applying it to an emotion that comes and goes like a passing cloud or a rain shower. The tyranny of words and our lack of discrimination have limited our development of true Love. Of course, I do not dispute that there is great value in even the emotion that we call love, although it should be more appropriately called liking or attraction. However, the danger is when we confuse this emotion with true Love, it can lead to all sorts of illusions and suffering.

If we think that the Divine Love is like our emotional love, then we will project all sorts of conditions on Divine Love. Our emotional love requires a quid-pro-quo: if we love someone then we require them to love us back or show some appreciation, and if they don't, then we may rescind our love or even feel emotionally hurt, leading to a feeling of hatred for the former object of love. Does God only Love those who love Him back and hate those that don't? In our confusion, that is exactly what we have projected and that has been written in many a holy book – that we must love Her for Her to love us back.

In reality, Love is a divine attribute and not an emotion. It is constant and unchanging in its all-encompassing and time-demolishing power. Even a mother's love is but an shadow of this Love. In yoga, we are striving to develop this Love.

The quality of this Love is illustrated by the following story:
There was once an old yogi who lived in a cave near a village. He would come into the village and sit under a tree to tell inspirational stories. The villagers would bring him leftover food. They would also occasionally bring those who were sick to him and he would whisper a few words, touch them gently and they would be miraculously healed.

The yogi sometimes fell asleep and would start snoring while sitting under the tree. In the village was a gang of rowdy kids whose leader was an especially naughty boy who was the terror of the village, as he loved to play pranks on the grown-ups. The victims could not punish him because he was the village chief's son. The gang took great pleasure in tormenting the old yogi – they would throw stones at him when he fell asleep and sometimes he would be bruised all over when he woke up. One day, as was their usual custom, the boys were throwing stones at the sleeping yogi and as he opened his eyes, the leader threw a big stone that struck his left eye and blinded the old man. In spite of the blood and pain, the yogi merely smiled at the boy, shook his head, hobbled up and went back to his cave.

A few days later, the old yogi came back to the village with his left eye heavily bandaged, but smiling as usual. Immediately, the village chief came and prostrated himself at the feet of the yogi and begged for his mercy and help. The yogi gently inquired what service he could do for him and the chief tearfully replied that this son, the gang leader who had blinded the yogi had fallen sick and the village doctor had proclaimed that it was an incurable plague and they had taken the boy to the forest to die. The yogi gave the chief his blessing and assured him that the boy would recover. The yogi asked for a pitcher of water which he blessed and then told the father to give the boy to drink. Within an hour of drinking the water, the boy's fever, pain and sores had subsided and he was able to open his eyes. The whole village marveled at the yogi's compassion, for they felt sure that the sickness was some sort of punishment, but it was the karmic wheel of justice, not the yogi who had delivered the punishment. It was the yogi filled with Love that delivered the cure.

Unity In Plurality

Since the goal of yoga is unity with the One Divine, why do we need to utilize images, mantras and other aspects of different manifestations of the Divine such as Ganesha or Lakshmi?

If we can purify ourselves from all our desires and achieve awareness of the Divine, then we can practice a duality focusing on the One, with the eventual merging with the subject of Unity, when all duality ceases. However, in our current state of confusion, it is not possible to become aware of the non-Manifest Divine and so we must focus on a Divine manifestation. In fact, our karmic tendencies make it difficult to even focus on the awareness of a single manifestation of the Divine and so in this relative world, we must make use of the tools of duality. We need to invoke various manifestations per our needs to overcome the obstacles to yoga.

Different seekers will resonate with different forms of the Divine and there may not be a universal form that can satisfy everyone. Some will resonate with the Divine Father Shiva, others with the Divine Mother Shakti, yet others with the Divine Son, or with various functional aspects such as Lakshmi, Saraswati or Krishna.

There will be some seekers who will not find it comfortable to utilize any image of the Divine and will be satisfied with the intellectual concept of the Divine, whether as the creator of the universe or as their true Being-Self.

There will be also those who see no need for the Divine and seek the unity beyond all concepts. However, it is cautionary to consider that even thinking the word non-duality is a dualistic phenomenon – it is not possible to utilize any human language or mind-born thoughts to contemplate non-duality or an attributeless Divinity. Only in a state of pure awareness, without mind or thoughts can non-duality be experienced.

Whatever the predilection of the seeker, until we can reach our goal, there will be times when we need to make use of the tools of the relative world – this is the utilization of skillful means in order to attain to non-dual wisdom.

Focus on Mudra –
Ganesha Mudra For Heart Chakra

Hold the left hand in front of the chest with the palm facing outward. Grasp the fingers of the left hand with the right hand, which has the palm facing towards the body. Move the hands in front of the chest up to the level of the heart.

Exhale and pull the hands apart without releasing the grip, tensing the muscles of the upper arms and chest area.

Let go of the tension and inhale. This is one round. Repeat 6 times for a total of 7 rounds. Then place the linked hands on the sternum and repeat the mantra for Lord Ganesha three times.

Change hand positions with the right palm facing outward and left palm facing inward. Repeat the exhalation and inhalation 7 times and then once more place the hands on the sternum. Intone the mantra for Lord Ganesha aloud 3 more times.

Focus on the heart center in silence for a minute or two.

This mudra strengthens the heart muscles and stimulates heart activity in general, releasing tension in the area. It opens up the heart chakra and stimulates courage, confidence and openness in relationships.

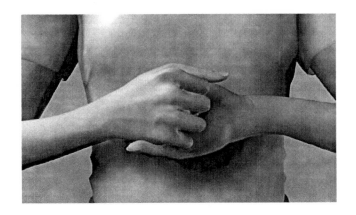

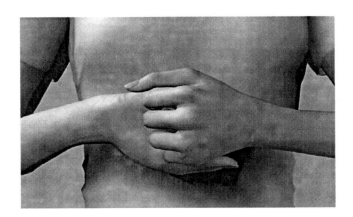

Figure 9: Ganesha Mudra

Yoga, Spirituality and Religion

A little while ago, I was discussing the goals and practice of yoga with a friend and it dawned on me that there was a lot of confusion concerning the spiritual path and the religious path, especially among those who are beginning the exploration into the spiritual but were brought up in traditional religious backgrounds. This situation is further obscured by the lack of agreement on what constitutes spirituality.

For many, the dichotomy is between spiritual and material and all knowledge and effort in the non-material plane is considered spiritual. A religion would then be considered spiritual as it appears to be concerned with concepts such as afterlife and God.

However, to those on a spiritual path such as yoga, religious systems seem to be anything but spiritual. The confusion is due to the fact that from time immemorial, there have been two approaches to the non-material – the majority are content with vague assurances of continuity after physical death and trust in the authority of someone or some organization to ensure happiness in the non-material realm while they themselves focus on getting some measure of happiness in the material world which they can experience.

The path of yoga is about experiencing the truths that have been taught for oneself in the present life. It is concerned with realization and not beliefs. The seeker must have faith in the yogic authority only as far as the wisdom needs to be relied on until one has achieved the same states described. As an analogy, if someone describes an attractive place for you to visit, you would have to rely on that description to motivate you to go there.

The path of yoga relies on individual practice to achieve the experience of the spiritual states described by the yogic guides and texts. This is similar to someone relying on a road-map to get to a destination – one must have faith in the accuracy of the directions to actually drive according to them. However, you must drive there yourself, rather than take a bus - analogies from material life can only be taken so far and do not apply fully!

Religion is a binding with rules and regulations, institutions, and hierarchies relying on blind obedience, threats of punishment and exclusivity. The believers do not usually have to make additional efforts beyond their agreement to join the group and subscribe to the same set of beliefs. If anyone should profess a deviant belief, that person would be branded a heretic. On the positive side, the believer is assured a place in heaven and can live a life unencumbered by other spiritual concerns.

Yoga is about expansion, freedom and openness to new experiences. However, one has to give up complacency and laziness. One has to take responsibility for one's own spiritual evolution. There is no free ride, no assurance of everlasting bliss without effort. On the plus side, one has the opportunity through hard practice to realize reality, overcome one's karmic chains, and to achieve freedom from the cycle of birth and death.

Yoga is not for everyone while religion is useful for the masses – each has its place in the schema of spirituality. In a more enlightened age nine thousand years ago, there was no religion or need for a separate yoga, the sages taught the Sanatana Dharma or Eternal Way. Perhaps in another five thousand years, humanity will be able to comprehend this vast teaching again.

We Need The Sun's Healing Energy Now

This is a time of transition. There is a breakdown in social and personal security. With increasing polarization and distrust among the nations and peoples, there is mounting violence and bloodshed in this fragile ecosystem we call Earth. A philosophy of peace, both world and personal, must be based on unity, rather than differentiation. It is now imperative that all of us understand the common bonds between all peoples. The great spiritual paths have all taught that the solution to the world's problems is to transcend the restrictive personal ego, and realize the higher dimensions of humanity - the essential one-ness underlying our individual experiences.

There is a common bond among all beings on earth. All life is based on and sustained by the great Light of the Sun. It is an indisputable scientific fact that there would be no life on Earth, without the Sun. Our Sun gives his life-force and light to all beings on earth, regardless of race, gender and beliefs. The rich and the poor are treated equally by the Sun. Those who act positively and those who act negatively are equally embraced by the light and love of this visible representation of the invisible Divine cosmic Love and Light.

There is no higher visible connection to the universal life-force then compassionate *Surya* [one of the many Sanskrit *Vedic* names of the Sun]. There is no greater source of healing and purification for humanity. Throughout the ages, all peoples have looked up to the Sun, in love and gratitude, for the gift of life. Some, propelled by dark ignorance, have distorted their 'worship' with self-serving and humanity-hating practices, while others have been led to ignore this visible representation of the invisible creator. It is a tragic fact that in no other time in humanity's past, have so many lost their connection with the

Sun, as we have.

It must be emphasized throughout that when the power of *Surya* is invoked it is not only the physical form of the Sun that is to be accessed, but the energetic and spiritual essence. Humanity has been endowed, not only with a physical form, but also with energetic, emotional, mental and spiritual aspects, and even plants have feelings. With what arrogance and ignorance do the children of the Sun, consider the creative agent, to be only an inert fireball?

When a spiritual seeker makes a connection with the Sun, she will heal the physical body, acquire greater vitality, overcome all negativity, and also come to a greater understanding and realization of her true nature.

The real nature and significance of the Sun has always been realized and taught by the true saints and seers of all cultures, especially by the ancient *yogis* of India. The great spiritual classics, such as Vedas and Upanishads all sing the praises of the Sun, the light, and the fire, as witness, friend and sustainer of all life. There is continuity from those ancient days to the current fast-paced, technologically driven culture – the Sun, Light and Fire are still praised everyday by millions in India. Tragically, much of the knowledge in other parts of the world have been lost or suppressed by neo-religious fanatics over the last several millennia.

Solar techniques and practices transcend and do not belong to any religion and are not religious practice in the usual narrow use of the term. However, they do help to open the practitioner up to a more profound and higher dimension of awareness and experience and are spiritual from that perspective. Regular practice will help one feel the unity and harmony of all life.

There is a trite, but nonetheless true saying that, "familiarity

143

breeds contempt," and sadly, humanity has often fallen prey to this fault in our psyche, and currently, even applied it to the greatest of beings in our solar system, the Sun. We no longer give thanks to the bringer and sustainer of life, and think ourselves superior to our ancestors, who stood in awe of manifest divinity.

The ancient *yogis* did not worship 'gods' as we now understand this concept. They sang in joy and gratitude to the Divine, which they "saw and experienced", as manifesting in different 'light beings' or *devas*. These ancient *rishis* in their cosmic enlightenment, sang praises to the principle of Light, by manifesting their unitary state in pluralistic thoughts, words and deeds, for the sake of seekers after the Truth.

These *Vedic* seers spoke in symbols of Light to awaken the internal Light in the heart of every being. To these Masters of life and death, the Sun or *Surya* is the symbol of the enlightened mind, the true Self, free from the darkness of ignorance.

Many names are used to describe the many aspects of the Sun, in the *Vedas*, and it is instructive to look at the meanings attached to some of these:

Surya:	Universal Soul, Great Witness
Savitar:	Creator, Great Transformer
Mitra:	Divine Friend
Varuna:	Infinite Space, Great Peace
Aditya:	Light
Vishnu:	Great Pervader
Pushan:	Great Sustainer

The *Sanatana Dharma* or Eternal Way, is the Solar transformation of darkness to light. The outer Sun is the visible representation of the inner light of transformation present in every human being.

For the Western World, the most defining time of the last

millennia, was the end of the 'Dark Ages', heralded by the efforts of Galileo and Copernicus, to put the Sun in its rightful place. Putting the Sun back in the center of our solar system started the Age of Enlightenment! Let us know begin the process of putting the Sun back in its rightful place in the center of our lives, and start the Age of Self-Realization.

We embrace the ultimate Bliss
Of the Divine Light, supporting all.
By holding our thoughts on Surya,
We reach the goal.

Rigveda 5.82.1

The Vedas For Today

The *Vedas* are the oldest source of knowledge and wisdom in the world, preserved by the people of India for thousands of years to represent their unbroken culture. The oldest of the *Vedas,* the *Rigveda* is now considered by impartial analyses to be between five and eight thousand years old. *Vedic* verses and mantras resound in homes and temples to the present day. They are not simply relics of the past but have inspired modern teachers to a new vision for the evolution of humanity.

The term *Veda* itself means knowledge, wisdom or vision, from the root 'vid' meaning to see or to know. This knowledge is considered in two levels, as a higher, internal or Self-knowledge, through which immortality can be gained, and a lower or external knowledge, through which we can understand the external world. The lower knowledge includes what the modern world refers to as science and technology.

Therefore, the *Vedas* should not be looked upon as religious documents only - they deal not only with ritual but also with *mantra* or the science of sound energy, *yoga* and meditation. They are source books for the deeper spiritual and mystical practices that lead to self-realization and cosmic consciousness, as well as for medicine, music, astronomy, cosmology, and architecture.

The *Vedas* emphasize experience, and are not books of blind belief and do not rest upon a person, institution or belief. They teach a path of knowledge that is open, and manifold. They are founded on the realization that there is One great truth behind the universe, a universal being and consciousness, but that it can be approached from many different levels and directions. The supreme principle of the *Vedas* is the Divine Self.

Meditation is taught as the way to true knowledge. The *Rigveda* recognizes a higher or meditative aspect of the mind, called 'dhi' as the faculty of true perception. From this same root 'dhi', the term *dhyana* for meditation arises. *Dhi* is the higher aspect of *manas* (mind), which enables us to perceive the eternal truth. This cultivation of *dhi* or *buddhi* is the main characteristic of Yoga, Vedanta and Buddhism.

Outwardly, the *Vedic* rituals consist of various tangible offerings, like wood or ghee, to the sacred fire, to generate a positive energy for the world. Inwardly, *Vedic* rituals consist of offerings of breath, speech and mind to the Divine or our higher Self to raise us to a higher consciousness and ultimate realization of our true nature.

Although there are thousands of *mantric* hymns in the *Vedas*, the number of hymns dedicated to specific divine principles are not necessarily reflective of their importance in the *Vedic* conceptual cosmos. There are only ten hymns specifically dedicated to *Surya* or the divine light within-and-without in the *Rigveda*, although some aspect of *Surya* is mentioned in many of the other hymns. The number ten is significant, because it is the number of completion.

Outwardly, *Agni* is the diety of the earth, while *Indra* is the diety of the atmosphere, and *Surya* is the ruler of the heavens. Inwardly, *Agni* is the individual soul or *jiva*, *Indra* is the *prana* or universal life-force, and *Surya* is *dhi*, or the light of consciousness. The union of *Agni*, *Indra* and *Surya*, is the union of the individual soul with the transcendental Self, to achieve the consciousness of light, truth and unity.

In the Vedas Self-Realization is the process of achieving unity with the divine Sun. The most often repeated mantra from the *Rigveda*, and the only one that appears in all the main Vedas, is the *Gayatri*, dedicated to *Surya-Savitar.*

Let us meditate on the brilliant light of the Creator,
the Sun,
to achieve inner understanding,
to illumine our intelligence,
to transform our earthbound consciousness
into the boundless Light of the inner Sun.

Spiritual Marriage

One of my dear students is getting married in a few days and while I'm thinking of her from afar, and wishing both the happy bride and groom the best, it is instructive to review the role of what would be considered a spiritual marriage. This is the same whether one formalizes it with a ceremony or it is an informal arrangement as it often is these days.

Spiritual seekers are often confused about the role of marriage on the spiritual path. Those who are unmarried are conflicted by their needs and social pressures versus their perception of the freedom to pursue their path. The married seekers are conflicted about their family duties versus their time alone for meditation and other spiritual pursuits.

Often the single seeker will look for a soul-mate with whom she can tread the path together, supporting each other with love and harmony. Whether this happens or not will depend on their karmic tendencies. There are also some practitioners who wish to scale the heights of higher consciousness on their own and believe that they can do so faster without a partner. There is no right or wrong as far as partnering or not is concerned – it depends on the balancing of karmic tendencies and one's dharmic role in life – that is to say, neither one is superior to the other and each person has to find their own way. It is one of the reasons I always counsel new students to get in touch with their higher intuition as soon as possible and provide the techniques for doing so – follow your heart and not your confused mind.

Often times, students come to me with their personal problems that include a marriage or relationship that has gone awry somehow. There are many instances where there is a divergence in their approach to spirituality. For example, the husband may be attracted towards yogic practices while the wife is a devoutly religious person believing in a personal savior and taught to denigrate a different approach from another culture. There are also cases where the materialistic husband opposes the wife's growing spirituality as it takes her away from his control. The common factors are differing beliefs, jealousy, fear, and control. Fear of losing a family member to some strange spiritual group often imperceptibly drives a wedge between loved ones. It is important to keep an open mind and cultivate harmony rather than conflict. Forcing someone else to share one's beliefs will not succeed in the long run for a health relationship.

In a traditional Indian marriage ceremony, there are many elements which are meant to teach the bride and bridegroom about how to live together in harmony with each one committing to make the relationship work, even if it means giving up something. However, it is important to remember that both partners must be willing to adjust from being single to living life as a partner, that is to say, both must be willing to change and work together – it cannot be one-sided.

A highlight of the ceremony is the **saptapadi** - marriage knot symbolized by tying one end of the groom's scarf with the bride's dress. Then they take seven steps representing nourishment, strength, prosperity, happiness, progeny, long life and harmony and understanding, respectively.

They make the following commitment to each other:

1. Let us stay together for the rest of our lives and may we be blessed with an abundance of resources and comforts, and be helpful to one another in all ways.

2. Let us not separate from each other and may we be strong and complement one another.

3. Let us discharge our prescribed duties to others and may we be blessed with prosperity and riches on all levels.

4. Let us be of one mind in carrying out our responsibilities and may we be eternally happy, achieving both material and spiritual wealth.

5. Let us love and cherish each other, enjoying nourishing food and good health and may we be blessed with a happy family life.

6. Let our aspirations be united – just like the melody and lyrics of a vedic mantra and may we live in perfect harmony... true to our personal values and our joint promises.

7. Let us respect each other even where we may not agree and may we always be the best of friends.

To point out the spiritual dimensions of the rite, there is the ***abhishek*** – a sprinkling of water for purification followed by meditating on the sun and the pole star which signify the spiritual portal and guide.

To demonstrate their mutual affection, there is the ***anna praashan*** - the couple make food offerings into the fire and then feed a morsel of food to each other expressing mutual love.

Towards the end of the ceremony, the husband lifts the wife and places her right foot on a flat granite grinding stone and recites the following:

As we stand on this firm stone, may our relationship be rock-solid.
Let us stand up to those who oppose us while we carry out our time-honored responsibilities as husband and wife as sanctioned by the wisdom and tradition.

Although I've updated the wordings of the ceremony to give a modern interpretation, it still retains the spirit of the original intent of the great Masters who gave us this traditional ceremony as guidance to a new phase on the path of a spiritual way of life.

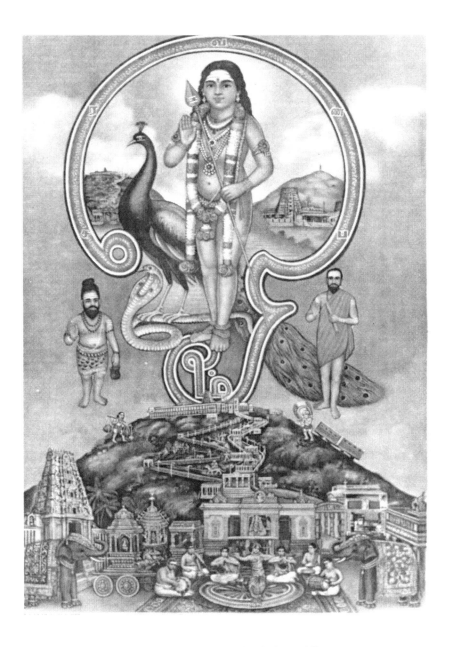

Lord Muruga: The Lord Of The Siddhas

More Books by Rudra Shivananda

Chakra self-Healing by the Power of Om
Breathe like your Life depends on It
Surya Yoga (out of print)
The Yoga of Purification and Transformation
In Light of Kriya Yoga
Healing Postures of the 18 Siddhas

For excerpts from these books and
purchase information:

http://www. alightbooks.com
http://www.amazon.com

About the Author

Rudra Shivananda is dedicated to the service of humanity through the furthering of human awareness and spiritual evolution. He teaches that the only lasting way to bring happiness into one's life is by a consistent practice of awareness and transformation.

Rudra Shivananda is committed to spreading the message of the immortal Being called Babaji. He teaches the message of World and Individual Peace through the practice of Kriya Yoga. A student and teacher of Yoga for more than 35 years, he is initiated by his Master Yogiraj Gurunath Siddhanath as an Acharya or Spiritual Preceptor in Kriya Yoga and the Indian Nath Tradition, closely associated with the Siddha tradition. He is also experienced as a Shakti Healer and Astrologer with expertise in the healing and spiritual uses of mantras, gemstones and essential oils. He lives and works in the San Francisco Bay area, and has given initiations and workshops in USA, Ireland, India, England, Estonia, Spain, Russia, Brazil, Canada, Japan and Australia.

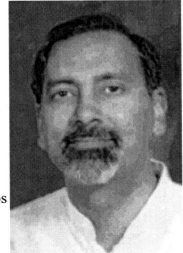

For informaton about his workshops and schedule:
www.rudrashivananda.com

LaVergne, TN USA
24 August 2009
155799LV00012B/92/P